PATIENT EDUCATION
A Practical Approach

Kate Lorig, R.N., Dr.P.H.

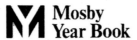
Mosby
Year Book

Dedicated to Publishing Excellence

Sponsoring Editor: Gayle Paprocki
Associate Managing Editor, Manuscript Services: Deborah Thorp
Production Manager: Nancy Baker
Proofroom Manager: Barbara Kelly

First Published 1991 in Australia and New Zealand by Fraser Publications
PO Box 1045, Ivanhoe, Victoria 3079, Australia

Mosby-Year Book, Inc.
11830 Westline Industrial Drive
St. Louis, MO 63146

1 2 3 4 5 6 7 8 9 0 ML 96 95 94 93 92

Library of Congress Cataloging-in-Publication Data

Lorig, Kate.
    Patient Education: A Practical Approach/Kate Lorig.
        p.   cm.
    Includes bibliographical references and index.
    ISBN 0–8151–5607–3
    1. Patient education.   I. Title.
    [DNLM: 1. Patient Education—methods   W 85 L872c]
R727.4L67   1991
615.5'07—dc20
DNLM/DLC   91–32515
for Library of Congress   CIP

PATIENT EDUCATION
A Practical Approach

with Kisses,
RN

Acknowledgments

Books don't just happen. This book is no exception. Over the years many people have been very helpful. Milton Chernin was the first to suggest that I might write a book. I regret I was too slow to allow him to see the finished product. Many people have helped me learn about patient education. These include Carol D'Onofrio, Wendy Cuneo, Larry Green, Rusty Rosenstock, Barbara Giloth, Sam Radelfinger, Helen Ross, Rosemary Pries, Kay Fox and Mary Hobbs.

For the past twelve years I have had three Stanford mentors and colleagues who have supported my work, tried to keep me on track and at the same time allowed me to explore uncharted territory. My very special thanks to Halsted Holman, James Fries and Albert Bandura.

Added to these professionals are the hundreds of people who have attended patient education workshops I have given in the United States, Canada, Australia, New Zealand and Sweden. You have asked important questions and have served as my guides for moving patient education from the ivory tower of academe to the clinical setting. In addition you have given me many ideas based on your practice.

Finally there is a group of friends and colleagues who have written, typed, proofread, edited, critiqued and in many other ways made this book more readable. My deepest appreciation to Diana Laurent, Virginia Gonzalez, Jean Goeppinger, Jane Howard-McKellar, Sheri Robinson, David Sobel, Bruce Campbell, Charles Watson, Jenny Davidson, Ian Fraser and last but not least, Dr Shapiro.

Preface

Many health professionals are attracted by the idea of patient education. Nurses, doctors, physical therapists, occupational therapists and others often come to realize that the long term value of treatment can be greatly enhanced if followed up by a program to increase compliance or to reduce the level of risk behavior.

The problem is that the well meaning efforts of people who try to run patient education programs are often rewarded with failure and disappointment. The main reason for this is not hard to guess: health professionals are highly skilled at providing specific kinds of therapy but have little or no background in planning and implementing education programs.

Many health professionals work on the basis that the simple provision of information will be enough to produce appropriate compliance or risk reduction behaviors. The truth is that the implementation of successful health promotion programs is a complex business that requires special skills. It requires at least a basic understanding of the process of health education and some knowledge of the modern literature on the subject. The trouble is that most clinicians do not want to spend an inordinate amount of time learning about health education.

Kate Lorig has attempted to bridge the gap between the academic literature on health education and the day to day needs of health professionals interested in setting up patient education programs. The resulting book is a happy compromise between the pragmatic and intellectual. Most important, it will certainly help health professionals get results from their efforts to carry out patient education.

Kate Lorig's book is well set out, and the very readable text effectively protects the newcomer from exposure to the detailed research on which the advice is based. At the same time, a professional health educator will find that the book gives a satisfying account of the modern literature on planning, implementation and evaluation of health education programs. It also provides a very useful 'bluffer's guide' to the theory of health education strategies.

In short, this is a welcome and practical handbook. It will markedly increase the probability that its readers will set up successful patient education programs and that they will be able to evaluate and document them with a minimum of fuss and effort.

Charles Watson, Health Department of Western Australia

Contents

Introduction

This book is designed to solve problems, give practical advice and build new skills. It is for health professionals who are not skilled in patient education, but need to know where to start and how to proceed. It may also be useful to students who are just beginning to learn the tricks of the trade. If used as a text, it will take you step by step through the process of conceptualizing, designing, implementing and evaluating patient education programs.

Over the past several years, I have been asked to give many patient education skills building workshops. Some of these have been sponsored by the Veterans Administration and the American Hospital Association in the United States, others by the Arthritis Societies of New Zealand and Canada, the Arthritis Foundations of various states in Australia and the Department of Rehabilitation at the University of Gothenburg in Sweden. Also, there were workshops for the Health Education Society in British Columbia and the Society for Public Health Education in Seattle, Washington.

During this same time, I have been running an arthritis patient education research project at Stanford University. This project has involved hundreds of community based courses for thousands of people with arthritis. Our research has shown that patient education can change behaviors, improve health status and save health care costs.

This book is a result of all the above activities. It is a collection of the bits and pieces designed for the workshops and reflects our experiences here at Stanford and the real life experiences of the workshop participants. Although there is a large section on health education theory, this is not primarily an academic book. Rather, it is my hope that the book will help practitioners use theory in everyday practice. In short, this is a 'how to' guide to patient education which grew out of my work over the past decade. I have tried to make suggestions which will have immediate relevance to practice. At the same time, many readers will want more information. Therefore, at the end of each chapter is a short bibliography so you know where to look next. Finally, I need help. If you have ideas to add or problems that are not mentioned, then please write. I'll incorporate your ideas in the next edition.

Some Words and Definitions

Now, a short discussion about words and definitions. Throughout this book,

I'll talk about 'patient' education. The reason for using the word 'patient' is that this is *not* a book about health promotion or disease prevention, although much from the book could be applied to such programs. Rather, it is about 'patients'—people who have a defined health problem, be it high blood pressure, cancer, diabetes or AIDS. Usually, when someone is receiving medical care for a condition, we call them a patient. This is especially true in hospitals and clinics. However, this same person with his or her illness is often found getting on with life in the community. In this case, he or she becomes a person with diabetes, high blood pressure, AIDS or whatever. Somehow saying education for people with _____ is rather awkward. Thus, for literary purposes and to save trees, I'll talk about patient education.

So now that we know what a patient is, let us define patient education. This is any set of planned, educational activities designed to improve patients' health behaviors and/or health status. Notice, there is nothing in this definition about improving knowledge. Activities aimed at improving knowledge are patient teaching. Changes in knowledge may be necessary before we can change behaviors or health status. However, just because someone has correct knowledge does not mean he or she will change. If all we needed was knowledge, we would have no smokers, overweight people or people eating high cholesterol foods. Patient education is much more than knowledge change.

The purpose of patient education is to maintain or improve health, or in some cases, to slow deterioration. The means by which this occurs are changes in behaviors and/or mental attitudes. Such things as increased compliance with medication taking, decreased pain, shorter hospital stays or decreased depression are all reasonable expectations for patient education programs.

Now that we have defined 'patient' and the purpose of patient education, there is one part left—'planned educational activities'. Patient education does not just happen. It is planned. This book is about the planning of patient education activities.

Kate Lorig, 1000 Welch Road, #320, Palo Alto, CA 94304

How to Use This Book

Being a patient educator is a little like being a Jack or Jill of all trades. Often you are called upon to design something such as a program or a one to one intervention. Other times you are asked to fix something. 'Why don't people come to my program?', or 'Why don't the patients do what I tell them to do?' Still other times, you are asked to evaluate patient education. Another role is that of supplier of resources. 'Where do I get information on Parkinson's disease?' or 'Where can I get a slide projector?' Sometimes you are expected to put all of these roles together and create, implement, and evaluate an entire program. This book is designed to assist you with all these roles. Each chapter is aimed at a specific function or problem. In the last chapter are an overview and some checklists to help you put the bits and pieces together into a recognizable whole. Unlike most books, this one does not need to be read beginning to end. Instead, there are several ways you get started.

- Like any other book, start with the table of contents and read what you want.

- Start with the following problem list. The chapter numbers after the problem show where you find answers.

- Start with the checklist on program planning found on pages 139–141. Again, the page numbers following each item indicate where it is discussed.

- As you read you will find page numbers for more information on related subjects.

All of this is to say that there are many roads to a good patient education program. Start wherever you feel best.

Problems

1 Doctors won't:
   Participate. *Chapter 4*
   Refer. *Chapter 4*
   Do what I want them to do. *Chapter 4*
2 Patients aren't motivated. *Chapters 1, 4 & 6*
3 Patients won't come. *Chapter 4*

How Do I Know
What Patients
Want and Need?

NEEDS ASSESSMENTS

Programs for educating patients do not just happen. Rather, they are built, based on the beliefs and skills of those offering the education. All programs start with someone believing that patients should know or do something. The program is then formed to see that this happens. The foundations of all programs are based on these initial beliefs. However, the strength of the foundation and therefore the whole program is determined by how well the program fits the needs of those it will serve. Unfortunately, unaided, health professionals are usually not able to fully understand patient needs. Therefore, many programs fall short. Solid patient education programs are built on carefully executed needs assessments. In this chapter, we will discuss six methods of conducting patient education needs assessments.

Interested Party Analysis

One of the most common problems in planning any new program is not considering the needs of all those involved. While it is evident that client needs are important, we often forget the needs of the other interested parties. For patients, there are often many such persons, including the patient, family, health professionals, friends, neighbors and other service agencies. Once the general topic of a program has been determined, i.e., cancer, diabetes or AIDS, it is important to make a list of all the interested parties.

The next step is to interview the key people to find out what they want from your program and how this program may impact on other programs. For instance, the fund raising branch of the organization may see the program as a source of new donors or of special interest to a new donor community. On the other hand, there may be concern with advertising for your program at the same time they are pursuing another large public campaign. Furthermore, the volunteer recruiter may be overwhelmed by the need to recruit and train an additional forty volunteers or may be overjoyed because your program will serve as a new recruiting tool. The assessment may have shown a need to provide services to a special language or cultural group. However, agency administration may be concerned that this would necessitate the hiring of bilingual staff, which could affect the budget.

Other agencies in the community may also have an interest in your plans. A program to assist the adult children of aging parents may be offered by other organizations or health providers. Your agency may find itself in a turf battle which could lead to unfavorable publicity.

Finally, the needs of clients and their families may be varied. Children undergoing chemotherapy may see teasing by peers as a major problem. Thus, the agency could provide a teasing inoculation program by training parents how to help their children. However, this program completely ignores the needs of parents of children with cancer, who must deal with family stress and the fear of future prognosis. Since most health problems affect not only the individual but also the family and community, it is important to get input from everyone before deciding the program focus.

The following is a suggested interview or questionnaire format for an interested party analysis. Remember, it is not etched in stone and is offered as a guide for you to change and use as you wish.

1   Name...

2   Reason for interviewing ....
    (For example, is this person a patient, family member, agency
    administrator, etc.?)

3   We are considering starting a..
    program and would be interested in your opinions.
    As a...
    your ideas are very important.

4   Considering your position, what do you think should be the
    objectives of the program? (For clients and their families, this
    question can be rephrased to, 'When you think of
    ...., what do you think of?')

5   What advantages do you see in starting this program?

6   What are the disadvantages or other possible problems that
    you foresee?

7   How do you see yourself (your agency) participating in this
    program?

8   Do you have any other thoughts that you would like to share
    with us?

You may want to ask other things during this same interview, such as best format, place, time, or how to fund the program. However, these questions are not necessary in the needs assessment stage and are sometimes best left until you know exactly where you are going.

Checklist Needs Assessment

Probably one of the most common forms of needs assessment is a questionnaire checklist. All you do is list a number of topics and let potential participants check off topics of interest. There are many advantages to this method. Checklists are easy to administer, clients seldom object, and they are also easy to tally. However, checklists should not be used as the sole means of getting information. The problem is that a checklist usually reflects what professionals are ready to teach, not necessarily the interests of the patients. For example, there are many checklists about cardiac problems that include such things as exercise, diet, medication, etc., but fail to mention the problems of living with uncertainty. We know from studies that uncertainty is usually a major concern for those patients. Why is it forgotten? Because living with uncertainty is not the central focus of any one health profession, and therefore sometimes falls through the cracks.

Many checklists do have an 'other' space. However, seldom are there enough similar 'other' responses to make these an important program planning consideration. All is not lost. Checklists can be useful if carefully constructed. The topics to be included should come from both patients and professionals. Focus groups are sometimes useful in writing checklists. See page 9. Be sure not to change the patient generated items, for example, changing 'living with uncertainty' to 'frustration'.

All in all, it is probably best not to rely solely on checklists. However, if you do, be sure to follow the above guidelines.

Salient Beliefs Assessment

From psychology, we learn that human beings can have only seven or so beliefs or opinions about any one subject. These have been called 'salient beliefs' (Miller, 1956; Fishbein & Ajzen, 1975). If you can identify these beliefs, you can then use this knowledge as a basis for your educational efforts. Assessing salient beliefs is especially good for the busy health care provider to use in one on one situations. A very simple way of soliciting these beliefs is to ask the client 'When you think of———, what do you think about?' The blank can be filled in with any behavior or disease (e.g., exercise or cancer). The answers that you get will give you good insight into that person's beliefs and concerns about that particular condition or behavior.

People with arthritis most often answer the above question with 'pain, disability and depression'. Knowing this, the health educator can then build a group or individual teaching program around pain management and preventing disability. If the patient's first response is fear, then the teaching should aim at determining the reason for the fear and trying to overcome it.

The above is one example of how the salient belief assessment can be used in one on one teaching. It can also be used as the basis for a group program. Here, a number of people with a similar condition or problem are asked, 'What do you think of when you think about——?'. They are asked to write as many answers to the question as they wish. These answers are then rated, with the first answer getting 10 points, the second answer 9 points, etc. The total score is then added for each response. The responses with the highest scores are the most important for that group. The following is an example of how to do this scoring:

Question: 'What do you think of when you think of menopause?'

Mary	Score	Jane	Score	Rebecca	Score
hot flushes	10	sagging body	10	fatigue	10
growing older	9	no birth control	9	hot flushes	9
no menstruation	8	dry vagina	8	getting old	8
loss of sex appeal	7	fatigue	7	fatigue	6

Scoring

Hot flushes	$10 + 9 = 19 \div 3 = 6.3$
Growing older	$9 + 8 = 17 \div 3 = 5.7$
No menstruation	$8 \div 3 = 2.7$
Loss of sex appeal	$7 \div 3 = 2.3$
Sagging body	$10 \div 3 = 3.3$
No birth control	$9 \div 3 = 3$
Dry vagina	$8 \div 3 = 2.7$
Fatigue	$6 + 7 + 10 = 23 \div 3 = 7.7$

Priorities for Teaching

Fatigue	7.7
Hot flushes	6.3
Growing old	5.7

Please note: These data are fictional and do not necessarily represent what should be taught about menopause.

One of the advantages of this technique is that it enables you to tailor the education to the perceptions and needs of the patients. For example, most traditional cardiac rehabilitation education does not directly address uncertainty, but focuses on exercise, medication and diet, which are the major concerns of health professionals working with coronary disease. These topics are all very important, but may be better accepted by patients if taught in the context of being better able to live with uncertainty.

A third way of using a salient belief assessment is when giving public lectures. Often we are asked to come and talk to a group about one topic or another. Since this is a one shot song and dance, we generally show a film or give a lecture. Rather, we might start the presentation by saying something like, 'When talking about AIDS there are lots of things we could say, such as what it is, who can get it, how do you get it, what is safe sex, how do you prevent it, etc. Before beginning, I want to know what you would like to know about AIDS. I will make a list and then we will vote on how you would like me to use my time.' At this point, ask the audience what they would like you to address. Write down all the items without comment and then read the list. Next, give everyone two or three votes and go through the list having the audience vote. Finally, address your talk to the top three or four items on the list.

This technique has several advantages. First, it involves the audience and lets them know that you are really interested in their input. Second, it allows you to address the issues of special interest to that group. One reason that some speakers are afraid to try this technique is that they think the audience will ask something that they are not prepared to address. Of course this can happen, in which case all you have to do is say that you don't know anything about how monoclonal antibodies affect AIDS and go on to the next topic. Most of the time, however, the topics chosen by the audience will be well known to you.

Matrix Assessment

This technique is especially good with a small group of no more than fifteen or twenty people. It is a quick variation on nominal group process or on the Delphi process (McKillip, 1987). First, ask everyone to write a list of what he or she would like to learn in the class. Make it clear that these lists are for reference only and will not be turned in. Have a large blank matrix like the one in Example 1.

Ask the first person to read his or her list. Put each item in a column space at the top of the matrix, and his or her name in the first row at the side of the matrix. Then put an X by each item in his column. Put the name of the second person in the next row. Put an X by all the items that he or she names for which there are headings at the top. Then add any new items to the column and add X's in an appropriate column. Continue this process for each person in the group. After everyone has exhausted his or her list, ask if anyone wants to add any X's anywhere on the matrix. It may be that some of the ideas of later people appeal to the earlier people. Finally add all the Xs in each row. The topics with the most Xs are the topics of most interest and should be emphasized. This process also allows all the participants to see how their interests fit with the others in the group. If there is one person with very different interests, he or she may decide that this is not the appropriate group or may decide to stay without expectations of having his or her specific interests met.

Example 1. Matrix Assessment Chart for a 'Stroke Club'

	How To Overcome Disabilities	Choosing A Doctor	Speech Problems	Controlling High Blood Pressure	Nutrition	Smoking	Stress Management	How To Choose A Nursing Home
John	X	X	X	X				
Maria		X	X	X	X		X	
Debbie	X				X	X		
Stan	X	X		X				
Pat		X					X	
Moses	X			X		X		
Joan		X			X			
Sasha	X	X		X				
Barbara	X				X			X
Jim	X	X					X	
TOTAL	**7**	**7**	**2**	**5**	**4**	**2**	**3**	**1**

Focus Groups

A fifth way of conducting needs assessments is to get together a small number of potential clients. Eight to twelve is an ideal number (Breitrose, 1988). It is important that the participants in the focus groups are like the people you are trying to reach. Focus groups usually work best if participants are similar. Thus, if you are trying to reach a very mixed audience, you might have several focus groups: one for the elderly women, another for the middle aged men, yet another for members of an ethnic minority community. Start by asking participants about their opinions. The secret is to be as non-directive as possible. For example, you might start by conducting a matrix assessment and then ask the focus group participants to discuss in more detail exactly what they would like to learn.

Another way to use a focus group is following a questionnaire. For example, you learn that stroke patients would like an exercise video tape for home use. A focus group could then be used to determine types of exercise desired, length of tape, willingness to buy the tape, etc.

Brainstorming can also be used to start a focus group. For more information, see page 41.

Focus groups can be used for program redesign. After a program has been given several times, a focus group of participants can often give insight into strengths and weaknesses. Focus groups can also be very helpful in suggesting new content or formats.

It is usually best to conduct a focus group with two people. One person actually conducts the group while the other keeps very careful notes. Of course, a tape recorder can be used instead of a note taker. However, this sometimes inhibits participation. Also, tape recorders and other mechanical devices have a nasty habit of having dead batteries or breaking the tape just when you need it most. When using any mechanical device, always have a back-up plan.

Structured Interviews

A final way of conducting needs assessments is through a structured interview. For this you make up an interview format similar to the example used for interested parties (see example, next page). A group of people like those you are trying to reach are all interviewed using the same format. These interviews can be done in person or by phone. Public opinion polls are good examples of the use of structured interviews.

This type of assessment is good in that, like the checklist, it is easy to administer and tally. In addition, you have the opportunity to clarify anything you don't understand. The disadvantage, like the checklist, is that you will never discover concerns which the interview doesn't cover. One way to get around this is by adding some open-ended or salient belief questions to your structured interview. If this is done, the open-ended questions should come before the structured questions. This helps avoid getting the answers the participants think you want to hear.

Example
Structured Interview

❏ When you think of diabetes, what do you think of? ....
  (Note: this is a salient belief question.)

❏ What are your greatest problems in living with diabetes? ....

❏ Would you attend a six-week class on diabetes? ....
     If yes, where should it be held? ....

❏ What times are best for you? ....

❏ What topics would you like covered? ....
     If no, how would you like to learn about diabetes? ....

❏ What would you like to know? ....

❏ What else about your diabetes would you like to tell us? ....

There is one note of caution in using needs assessments. If you already know what you are going to do and have no intention of changing, do not conduct a needs assessment. Nothing makes people angrier than being asked their opinions and then having those opinions ignored.

In conclusion, we have examined several ways of conducting needs assessments. There are also many other ways, including surveys, attitude-behavior-belief scales, and sampling. There is no one right or wrong way. Rather, you should use the method or methods which best fit your situation and will give you the information you need to know.

Patient education is not a science. There is no exact formula. It is an art and, as such, it is up to you to mix and match methods to achieve the best program for your situation.

Questionnaires on Computer

The preparation and analysis of questionnaires can be made much easier by the use of a public domain software product called EpiInfo. This program was written at the Centers for Disease Control (CDC) in Atlanta, Georgia, and was originally intended for the use of public health officials investigating outbreaks of infectious disease. Despite its specialized beginnings, EpiInfo is a versatile tool for the preparation of questionnaires of all kinds. Answers to questions can be entered on the computer and automatically added to a database. The resulting information can be analyzed with a variety of statistical tests and can be printed out in tabular or graphical form.

EpiInfo includes its own word processor but questions can be prepared on standard office word processing programs and transferred to EpiInfo. Questionnaire data can be exported to other spreadsheet, database or statistical analysis programs (such as SPSS).

Perhaps the best thing about EpiInfo is that the software program is free. You can legally copy both the program disks and the manual. However, you can also order an original copy of the disks and manual from a distribution company acting on behalf of CDC. The latest version (EpiInfo 5) costs about $35 and can be ordered from USD Inc., 2156-D West Park Court, Stone Mountain, GA 30087, telephone (404)469-4098.

References

1 Breitrose, P.,
 Focus Groups - When and How to Use Them: A Practical Guide,
 Stanford University, Palo Alto, Calif, Health Promotion Resource Center, 1988.

2 Fishbein, M. Ajzen, I.,
 Belief, Attitude, Intention and Behavior, Reading, Mass., Addison-Wesley, 1975.

3 McKillip, J.,
 Need Analysis: Tools for the Human Services and Education.
 Applied Social Research Methods Series, Sage, vol. 10, 1987.

4 Miller, G.A.,
 The Magical Number Seven, Plus or Minus Two: Some Limits on Our Capacity for Processing Information, *Psychological Review,* 631:81-87, 1956.

CHAPTER 2

Do You Know Where You Want to Go?

And Will You Know
When You Get There?

EVALUATION

When you have examined the first step of developing a patient education program needs assessment, your second step, though not intuitive, is evaluation. In planning a good program, evaluation must be considered early. It is an important step in clarifying program goals. All too often, evaluation is an afterthought, not an integral part of program planning. This chapter will examine the questions to ask, types of evaluations, and evaluation design. By considering evaluation early, you can avoid problems and shape your program towards the outcomes you are trying to achieve. Let's look at some examples.

❑ EVALUATION AS AN AFTERTHOUGHT:
I wonder if our stop-smoking program was successful. We know that one year after the program we had a 30% quit rate. However, we don't have a control or comparison group (we just didn't think about it soon enough). Therefore, we don't know if 30% is good or bad. (In fact, this is an average or better one year quit rate.)

❑ EVALUATION AS AN AFTERTHOUGHT:
I sure would like to ask the mothers who came to our children's health fair what they found most useful. Unfortunately, I don't have any way of contacting them. In fact, I don't even know who came—just how many.

❑ EVALUATION AS AN AFTERTHOUGHT:
I wonder if people who were referred to our weight loss program by doctors lost more weight than those who answered advertisements in the newspaper? However, I don't know how people learned about the program.

Asking the Right Questions

In any evaluation, the most important part is asking the right questions. All evaluations start with the same two questions: (1) What do you want to know? and (2) Who cares? Or put more nicely: What difference does it make? It is very important to spend a great deal of thought and time answering these two questions. As soon as you start to do an evaluation, you will think of a million things you would like to know. Then, just to complicate matters, all your colleagues will think of extra things that they would like to add to your evaluation. The result can soon become a

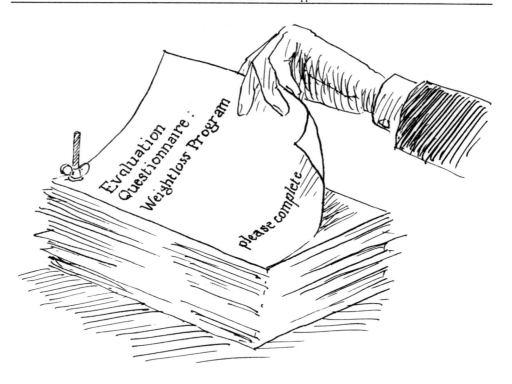

three hour interview or a fifty page questionnaire. Stop! Decide three to five things that are the goals of your program and that you *most want* to know. Stick with these. There are several problems with collecting lots of data. First, the longer the evaluation, the fewer are the people who will complete it. Second, when you are finished you are likely to be swimming in data, and will not have enough time to analyze everything you have collected. In short, use the KIS principle – Keep It Simple.

Once you have more or less decided the questions you want to ask, put them to the acid test. Ask yourself, Who cares? If you cannot give a clear concise answer without beating around the bush, you probably don't have very good questions. By the way, when your colleagues come up with extra questions, you can use the same test. Ask them, Who cares? As a rule of thumb, if an interview or questionnaire takes more than fifteen minutes to complete, it is probably too long. (Please note, this is not true when doing research as opposed to program evaluation.)

Types of Evaluation Questions

There are generally two types of evaluations: process evaluation and outcome evaluation. Of course, it is possible to do both at the same time.

However, you need to be clear about what you are doing. Process evaluation, sometimes known as formative evaluation, involves finding out what is going on with your program. The types of questions asked are: How many people came? Did the leaders follow the protocol? What questions were asked? Where did people find out about the program? What did the program cost? How did people like the program? What did they not like? Were the instructors comfortable with the material? How many telephone calls did our advertisement generate?

Outcome or summative evaluation does just what it says. It examines if the program accomplishes what it set out to accomplish. Did participants have lower blood pressure, were they hospitalized less, did they stop smoking or change other health behaviors, are the doctors being asked more questions? Sometimes there is a fine line between process and outcome evaluations. For example, in these days of great competition among health care plans and providers, health education is often seen as a marketing tool. Thus, you might do an outcome evaluation to see if a large-scale community health education program resulted in greater awareness of the plan or more satisfaction with the plan. These are not generally considered health education outcomes. However, they are very acceptable outcomes for a marketing program. Again, the important thing is to be clear about what you are doing and why you are doing it. There is nothing wrong with participating in a marketing program as long as there are also some health education objectives.

As we said earlier, evaluations can clarify program goals and even suggest program implementation strategies.

Methods: How Do I Find Out What I Want to Find Out?

As with types of evaluation, there are two basic evaluation methods: qualitative and quantitative. Some people might label these as subjective and objective evaluations. Don't get caught in this trap! There is nothing inherently subjective or objective about either method, nor is one method better than the other. Rather, the best evaluations use both methods. The question, not the bias of the evaluator, should be the basis for your choice of evaluation method.

Qualitative Evaluations

Qualitative methods are often used for answering 'messy' questions. Sometimes we want to know why something happened: for example, why heart disease patients stopped smoking. One way of getting the answer is to make a list of all possible reasons and have the ex-smokers check off the answers. The problem here is that no one can make an all-inclusive list. You will only get the answers on your list and may miss the real reason that people stopped smoking. In this case, using qualitative methodology would probably be better. Just ask people why they stopped smoking. Then have three judges read all the answers and form a list of general categories. Compare the three lists of categories and form one list of categories. You should not have more than ten or twelve categories in all. Now go back through all the answers and have each of the three judges fit every answer into a category. Finally, compare the category placement of the three judges. Hold a discussion until consensus is reached for any differences in opinion. If some responses don't fit a category then form new categories. It is important that all responses fit a category. An 'other' category doesn't count. Also, it is important that consensus is reached where there is a disagreement.

Now you may think that this would be much easier if only one person did all the above steps. You would certainly avoid disagreement. While this is true, you might also miss some of the most important material. For example, when doing a study of the problems of handicapped children in school, the children often mentioned problems with physical education courses. Two of the judges put these responses into a category of physical problems. However, the third judge, who had been a handi-capped child, put these responses into the social problems category. She ultimately convinced the other two judges to agree with her. As you can see, the solution to this problem is very different depending on whether you consider it a physical or social problem.

Generally, qualitative evaluations take more time than quantitative ones. However, they often result in perspectives which would have been lost if only quantitative data had been collected. Incomplete perspectives can lead to weak programs. For example, one evaluator doing a study of compliance asked cardiac patients how often they forgot to take their medications. She concluded that patients forgot 20 to 40% of the time, so she built a program based on memory aids. Another evaluator asked cardiac patients why they didn't always take medications as directed, and found that medications were missed in social situations. They were also missed because of misinterpretation of symptoms. The patient felt better and therefore decided there was no need for the medication, felt worse and decided the medication was not helping, or suffered side effects and decided not to take the medication. Using these findings, the second evaluator based her program around rehearsal of medication taking in social situations and reinterpretation of symptoms. It is most likely that the second program will gain greater compliance than the first.

In choosing between quantitative and qualitative evaluations, a good rule to follow is that if you are not sure what you need to know, use qualitative methods. Ask the people who know, usually the patients.

Very often when conducting evaluations you ask questions of the wrong people or maybe not of enough categories of people. For example, sometimes you want to know why people drop out of classes or have very sporadic attendance. To find the answer you often ask the instructors. Now everyone always has a very legitimate reason for not coming to class—an aunt is visiting, they went on vacation, a child was sick, etc. Unless people are very angry, they will never tell the instructor that they were bored, the room was uncomfortable, or that their classmates had bad body odor. Thus, if you want to find out why people dropped out, call them and ask. A few carefully worded, tactful questions over the phone can get you heaps of information.

One last point about asking qualitative questions. Experiment a little with wording. Remember that people don't generally like to be negative. Therefore, asking what participants did not like about the program will not get much information. Rather, ask what they would change in the program. Also, if you ask what people liked, the answer is often 'everything'. Again, this is not a very helpful answer. Instead, ask 'If you could attend only two or three parts of this program, what would you choose to attend?' This type of question forces participants to make a choice without being obnoxious. If you don't know how to ask a question, ask it three or four different ways and see which way yields the most useful (note, I did not say the best) answers.

Quantitative Evaluations

Most evaluators favor quantitative evaluations or those which collect numbers. To begin with, these are generally easier to conduct and somehow numbers seem more solid than opinions. In some cases, this is true and in others it is not. You would not ask someone to give you their opinion about their blood pressure reading: you would take their blood pressure. On the other hand, as we have already seen, valuable data are often lost in quantitative evaluations.

Usually, quantitative evaluations are conducted using a questionnaire, clinical data or data which have already been collected for something else. Let us look at the last first. Suppose that you want to conduct a hypertension program and want to know how many hypertensives there are in your institution. You might take the blood pressure of everyone who walks in the door for a week. This would give you some idea. An easier approach would be to go to the pharmacy and find out how many prescriptions are given out for hypertensive medications during the week. Both of these data collection methods have many flaws. However, as can be seen, one is much easier than the other.

You will generally end up collecting your own data. This is usually done by use of a questionnaire. Questionnaire design is both an art and a science. One rule is, whenever possible, do not make up your own questions. A tried and true scale exists for almost anything you want to know: disability, depression, attitudes toward self care, helplessness, quality of life, coping strategies, etc. Your job is to find the correct scale. Start by going to the library and find out how others have measured what you want to measure. Read articles on scales or read articles on similar patient education programs and see how they were evaluated. The journals *Patient Education and Counseling* and *Behavioural Medicine Abstract* are excellent sources of such articles. Once you have found the names of one or two researchers who are interested in the same thing you are, write them a letter or call them up. These researchers spend their lives using and constructing questionnaires. Therefore, they can probably point you to the best instruments for your purpose. Don't be shy — most researchers are happy to share their knowledge with practitioners. Another source of help may be your local university or college. If there is a health education program, start there. Doctors or nurses interested in health services research or education can also be helpful, as can people in psychology departments. Use your community resources and you will save yourself a lot of time and effort. One word of caution: researchers may overwhelm you with more information and details than you want. Remind them, in a kindly way, that you are not doing research, you are evaluating a program and need to start in an easy straightforward manner. To help you we have included several helpful questionnaires in Appendix 1.

Once you have chosen your questionnaire, you have to get it filled out and returned. Again, this is not as simple as it sounds. The following table was adapted from the work of Ruth Fleshman, and may help you avoid some of the questionnaire pitfalls (Archer & Fleshman, 1985).

WHAT CAN GO WRONG WITH QUESTIONNAIRES—AND USUALLY DOES!

AILMENT	POSSIBLE REASON	POSSIBLE SOLUTION
They don't return the form.	Takes too much effort to get it back.	Make it easier. Send a stamped envelope. If local, make the return point as central as possible or pick them up yourself. Send a short, friendly letter explaining the study and encouraging their quick response.
They didn't even do them!	People have a right not to participate.	Accept it or remind them with a postcard or phone call.
	May not be as interested in the topic as you are.	Jazz it up. Try to increase their motivation to participate.
	Didn't understand what you wanted.	Call to get responses to a few important questions. Keep things as clear as possible—people don't struggle to understand. It's just easier to throw it away. Provide an example response. Really good pretests would have shown a problem here.
They didn't answer all the items.	Not time enough.	Don't rush them. Call them. Don't ask too many questions for the time allowed or for the effort it takes.

WHAT CAN GO WRONG WITH QUESTIONNAIRES—AND USUALLY DOES!

AILMENT	POSSIBLE REASON	POSSIBLE SOLUTION
They left an answer blank.	Maybe some were uncomfortable to answer.	Try to eliminate unnecessary sensitive items.
		Try wording uncomfortable items to carefully minimize the reaction.
		May not be able to get at crucial stuff in the way; may need a relaxed, trusting interview.
	Maybe they didn't know what to answer; not enough information or had no opinion.	Be careful to ask items your sample could be expected to know
	Maybe you didn't give them the choice they wanted.	At least at pretest, and if possible at test, leave one space open for 'Other' (specify)
They cut off my secret identifying code.	People aren't as dumb as they used to be.	Be open with your identification. Ask them to sign; but it has to be voluntary. (You risk getting fewer returned.)
		Don't bank on knowing exactly who they are.
On follow-up questionnaires you can't find participants.	They moved away or are deceased.	On the first questionnaire, ask them to provide the name, address and phone number of someone who'll know their whereabouts in one or five years.
They marked too many answers.	Maybe the choices you gave weren't mutually exclusive.	If the choices are of the same kind, try to combine them into a single answer that reflects both parts.
	Questions and answers spaced too close together.	Sometimes you can figure out which is the most likely to answer.

WHAT CAN GO WRONG WITH QUESTIONNAIRES—AND USUALLY DOES!

AILMENT	POSSIBLE REASON	POSSIBLE SOLUTION
	Some answers depend on different circumstances.	Be prepared to have to jettison items or whole forms for those problems.
	Your directions were not clear.	Be sure initial directions and even each page or item say how many to mark.
		But some people just won't follow directions anyway!
They added their own answer.	Maybe you forgot a whole answer category.	Hope you can include that on the next go-round.
		It is better to get this on the pretest but you can't always be so lucky.
		Try to fit their answer within existing categories.
Everybody marked the same answer.	You picked a skewed sample.	Unless it's contraindicated, look for balance in other groups.
	You didn't break the answers down far enough.	Remove the item for reworking, retesting, etc.
	You asked an obvious question.	Dumb!
	You just confirmed a major trend.	Publish your finding fast.
I don't think they answered honestly.	May be hostile to tests, the situation, you, etc.	Try to win their cooperation.
		Be ready to toss out obvious goof-ups.
	May have a sense of humor, be drunk, etc.	Ditto.
	May be guarding confidential material.	If it is vital to know, use double items to check reliability.
		Be prepared to lose items.

WHAT CAN GO WRONG WITH QUESTIONNAIRES—AND USUALLY DOES!		
AILMENT	POSSIBLE REASON	POSSIBLE SOLUTION
		Try to figure out why they'd want to lie and judge what to do accordingly.
		The bottom line is trust people; they usually tell the truth.
Why didn't I think to ask just that one other question?	Even researchers aren't omniscient!	Try a new form. Set up a dummy conclusion as completely as you can *before* you give the test; using your imagination this way can often suggest an omitted item.
		Try a new group with it added.
		Better luck next time.
They took so long to return it.	You didn't put a return date on it.	Place the date by which you need it where it's sure to be seen.
		Send a reminder a week or so after the due date to remind those who have not yet returned them. (This is where it pays to know just whose identification.)

Remember, always be nice; the participant is always right.

Finally you have all your data. Now what to do? Data analysis and statistics usually make the eyes of a patient educator glaze. Don't become catatonic. First there are some good, easy to use statistics books for beginners (Ambrose & Ambrose,1977; Swinscow,1980). You might be surprised at what you can do yourself. Even without a statistics book, you can do averages and tallies. This may be enough. Thirty % of the people stopped smoking for one year. The average class attendance was 4.2 out of six sessions. Participants lost an average of five pounds during the ten week program.

Again data analysis is a place where you can get help. However, don't wait until the end of your project to talk with a statistician. The time to start talking is when you are beginning your evaluation. Statisticians are much more than numbers crunchers. If you get one interested in a project early, he or she can be a huge amount of help. Unfortunately, some statisticians don't speak English; they speak their own brand of professional jargon. If possible, avoid this type. By the way, you probably don't need a card-carrying statistician. Very often anyone with an advanced degree in one of the health sciences can help you.

Study Design

Like questionnaire design, study design is an art. There are several excellent books which will give you lots of good ideas (Windsor, Baranowski, Clark, Cutter, 1984; Green & Lewis, 1986). The most important thing to remember is that quantitative evaluations need some type of comparison. Participants can be compared after the program to how they were before the program. That is how we got the 30% quit rate for smokers. Sometimes participants are compared several times. For example, you get exercise rates four months before the program, when the program starts, four months later, eight months later and one year later. This is a time series design and has the advantage of letting you know two things. First, did your program cause the exercise or was it caused just by time? What you might find is that 20% of the group starts exercising in the four months before the program. However, after the program, 70% of the group is exercising. This suggests that the program is responsible for getting 50% of the group to exercise. By continuing to collect data you can find out how long program effects last. If at eight months only 10% of the population is exercising, then the program's effect didn't last very long. However, if at one year 50% of the people are still exercising, you know that the program had a good long term effect.

Usually, the strongest design is one which has a randomized comparison group. In this case, you would take all the people who were interested in a program and let half of them take the program while the other half were not allowed to take the program or were asked to wait for several months before taking the program. In this way you can compare those taking the program with those not taking the program. When the two groups are randomly chosen, they are probably very similar. Therefore, any effects that you find are likely to be caused by your intervention

25

and not differences in the groups.

Most health education practitioners are reluctant to use a randomized design because they are afraid that those told they cannot take the program will be angry. In reality we have found that if people understand what you are doing and why, they are usually quite willing to wait a few months for their education. In ten years at the Stanford Arthritis Center, we have had 2500 people participate in randomized studies where the controls have been asked to wait four to eight months. We have seldom had any problems either getting or maintaining the control group.

If a randomized comparison group is not possible, then it may be possible to find a similar but non-randomized comparison group. This could be hypertension patients from another hospital. Or you may want to give your program in one part of the city, using people in another part of the city as controls. In any case, the important thing to remember is that the comparison group must be as similar to the treatment group as possible.

The above discussion has been designed to give you a few ideas about the thought process that goes into any evaluation. You cannot become an evaluation expert overnight. Like anything else, evaluation is a skill. You need practice and guidance to become proficient. However, all practitioners can be good evaluators. Just don't be afraid to stick your toe into the water. You might find you even like swimming!

References

1   Ambrose, H.W., Ambrose, K.P.,
     A Handbook of Biological Investigation, Winston-Salem, N.C.,
     Hunter, 1977.

2   Archer, A., Fleshman, R. (eds),
     Community Health Nursing Patterns and Practice, Mass., Darbery
     Press, 1985.

3   *Behavioural Medicine Abstracts* published quarterly by the Society
     of Behavioural Medicine. For subscription information, write: SBN
     National Office, 103 S. Adams St., Rockville, MD 20850. (As of 1992
     this is combined with the *Annals of Behavioral Medicine*.)

4   Green, L.W., Lewis, F.M.,
     *Measurement and Evaluation in Health Education and Health
     Promotion*, Palo Alto, Calif., Mayfield, 1986.

5   *Patient Education and Counseling,* published quarterly in conjunction with the International Patient Education Council. For subscription information, write: Elsevier Scientific Publishers, Ireland Ltd, P.O. Box 85, Limerick, Ireland. (Each year publishes a list of literature reviews for many diseases.)

6   Swinscow, T.D.V.,
Statistics At Square One, London, British Medical Association, 1980.

7   Windsor, R.A., Baranowski, T., Clark, N., Cutter G.,
Evaluation of Health Promotion and Education Programs, Palo Alto, Calif., Mayfield, 1984.

CHAPTER 3

How Do I Get From an Idea to a Program?

PROGRAM PLANNING AND IMPLEMENTATION

Putting together a patient education program is a little like being a juggler. You have to keep several balls in the air at the same time. While the first ball is nearly always a needs assessment, the other balls are launched more or less simultaneously. At the same time you are considering how to evaluate your program, you should be launching the plan for its implementation. In other words, you will have to make lots of decisions about what your program will look like.

Special Problems With Groups

When patients come to groups, they come for different reasons and have different knowledge and skill levels. This is true no matter how specific you try to make your intake criteria. Therefore, in any group setting, meeting the needs of the individual members is a problem. There are several ways of handling this. First, make sure that all members know what to expect from the course. This can be done by use of a matrix needs assessment. See page 7. If you find that someone has very different needs than the rest of the group, you can let him or her know that this might not be the educational program for them. The outliers then have the option of staying or not. If they do stay, they will have no illusions about what the course will cover.

Another way of dealing with differences is to have everyone work on developing their own behavioral program. Thus, in teaching a class on lowering cholesterol, some people may choose to increase fiber, others to cut down on eggs and dairy products and still others to eat less red meat. When behaviors are flexible instead of prescriptive, they are much more likely to be meaningful. See page 32.

Finally, people with more knowledge and skills can be utilized to help those with less background. They can help in problem solving and can sometimes also be used as successful coping models. See page 114. It is important that group education avoid being too rigid and prescriptive. If it is flexible, the varied backgrounds of the participants become an advantage, not a problem.

Setting Priorities—Choosing What to Teach in the Time Allotted

Whether patient education is given in five, ten or fifteen minute blocks, or several hour-long classes, you never have enough time to teach everything. Thus it is necessary to set priorities. Making decisions about what to teach requires three steps:

❑ listing all behaviors affecting the particular condition

❑ determining which behaviors are most important in affecting health status

❑ determining which behaviors are the easiest to change given a limited amount of educational time.

Let us examine these three steps.

Listing Behaviors

For all health conditions there are a number of behaviors which, if changed, would affect the condition. For example, someone with hypertension might be advised to stop smoking, lose weight, cut down on sodium, exercise, reduce stress, and comply with medication usage. A similar list can be made for any condition. The first step in setting priorities is to make a list of all behaviors which might affect the condition.

Determining the Effectiveness of Each Behavior

This is probably the most difficult part of priority setting. As health educators, we do not know a great deal about the relative effectiveness of health behaviors on health outcomes. However, not all behaviors are equal. In lowering blood pressure, medication compliance and smoking cessation are probably the most important – with weight loss, sodium reduction, and exercise coming somewhere in the middle. Stress reduction, although very popular, probably has only a limited long term effect on hypertension. Therefore, in choosing priority behaviors, you should first look at smoking cessation and medication compliance.

The question arises: how do you determine the relative effectiveness? This is where you should use experts. Ask physicians or epidemiologists to help with this problem. You can also read the studies yourself. One important note of caution: do not set priorities based on the popular press. For example, recently, we have been urged to cut down on dietary cholesterol. There is no question that blood cholesterol affects heart disease and that, for someone with very high blood cholesterol, cutting down on dietary cholesterol may help. However, big changes in blood cholesterol usually require medication. Most of the major studies showing that lowering cholesterol has reduced heart disease have accomplished this primarily through medication usage. Our knowledge of the effects of lowering cholesterol through dietary means is much more fragmentary. This is especially true for the elderly. What does all this mean? Should we do nothing? No, we should continue to urge a low cholesterol diet, but also realize that this should not be at a cost of quality of life. The fad of today may well be seen as the mistake of tomorrow. Remember, twenty years ago we were urging everyone to eat red meat. In short, be responsible for knowing a little about the research base for those behaviors you are urging others to change.

Which Behaviors Are Relatively Easy to Change?

We all know that some behaviors are easier to change than others. For example, it is relatively easy to get someone to take a pill once a day and much more complex to get someone to get and keep his weight down. The next step is to look at the items you mentioned as being important to health and rank them as to how easy or difficult each is to change. Depending on the amount of time, you can now choose which behaviors are most appropriate for your program. If you have only ten minutes with a hypertensive patient, you might concentrate on medication compliance and lowering sodium intake. On the other hand, if you have ten hours, you might work on diet, exercise and smoking behaviors in addition to compliance and sodium reduction.

Another way of setting priorities is to let the patient choose. Make a list of all the things which someone might do. For example, to lose weight this list might include not eating after 7 pm, not eating between meals, broiling foods instead of frying them, cutting down on sweets, cutting down on fats, eating more fruit and vegetables, increasing exercise, etc. Then let the patients choose the behaviors which they feel they can accomplish. This method has two advantages. First, you do not have to tell the patient everything about dieting and exercise. If there is something on the list he does not understand, he can ask. Second, the patient is given choices and control. The more the new health behaviors are chosen rather than prescribed, the better the chance that they will be adopted.

In short, priority setting is based on the amount of time, the importance of the behavior and the ease with which the behavior can be changed.

Refining Your Content

Once you have decided on your target behaviors, the next step is to define what someone needs to know and what skills they must have to accomplish the behaviors. For example, patients with hypertension probably don't need to know the anatomy and physiology of the cardiovascular system. However, they do need to know the most effective ways to stop smoking and to remain non-smokers. They need skills in fending off the social pressures to overeat and smoke, and how to change the environmental cues for smoking and eating. One of the greatest errors in many patient education programs is to spend a lot of time on interesting 'facts' at the expense of learning and practicing necessary skills.

Sometimes refining content is almost self-evident. To comply with appropriate medication use, patients must know when to take the medication and how much to take. Often, to learn about necessary skills and knowledge, it is necessary to go to the literature. In many areas of patient education, including smoking cessation, dietary changes and exercise programs, there has been research on what patients need to know and do. You may have to juggle, but you don't have to recreate the whole circus*.

Setting Objectives

Once you have done your needs assessment and chosen your content, the next step is to write objectives. These objectives make clear what you are trying to accomplish and will serve as standards for evaluation. Just as there are two types of evaluations, there are two types of objectives.

❏ PROCESS OBJECTIVES are those by which you determine the process of the patient education. Examples are:

  ❏ Fifty people will receive diabetes education this year.

  ❏ Publicity for the program will appear in six newsletters.

  ❏ Each participant will speak at least once at each session.

  ❏ Some 70% of the participants will make a contract for at least one behavior change.

---

* Each February, *Patient Education and Counseling* publishes a list of patient education literature reviews.

Note that in writing process objectives we have said nothing about changing health behaviors or health status. Instead we have dealt with managerial and teaching process.

❏ OUTCOME OBJECTIVES are the second type of objectives. They tell what we hope to accomplish in terms of changes in health behavior or health status. Examples include:

   ❏ After two hours of instruction, 70% of the diabetics will be able to self-inject insulin.

   ❏ By the end of the course, 80% of the participants will report that they walk four or more blocks three times a week.

   ❏ After instruction, 60% of the patients will have a diastolic blood pressure below 90.

   ❏ Sixty % of the persons screened at the health fair and found to have a high cholesterol reading will see a doctor within one month.

Having seen some examples of process and outcome objectives, let us now examine how to write objectives. All objectives have three parts: (1) an action, (2) criteria for the action, and (3) a criterion for judging if the action has been accomplished.

An Action

The action or verb part of the objective must be something that you can hear or see. Sometimes you can also use smelling or tasting verbs. However, these are not always useful in patient education objectives. Words such as *report, eat, walk, have* a diastolic pressure, etc., are good action verbs for an objective. On the other hand, words such as *know, understand, think,* and *feel* are not good action words. There is no way that you can see someone 'knowing'. If your objective is that the participants will have more knowledge, then the objective should read, 'Eighty % of the participants will score 70 or above on a diabetes quiz.' Or, 'When asked to name their medications, 75% of the participants will be able to name all the prescription medications that they will be taking when they leave the hospital.' 'Participants will feel more in control of their asthma', is not a good objective. Rather, 'Eighty % of the patients will increase their score by ten or more points on an asthma self-efficacy scale.'

❑ CHOOSING THE ACTION

Probably the most important part of writing an objective is choosing the correct action. The question to ask yourself is, Who cares? It is all fine and good that patients score well on a quiz. However, we know that changes in knowledge do not necessarily lead to changes in behavior or health status. If they did we would have no smokers, alcoholics, over-weight people or people who do not floss their teeth. Thus knowledge objectives are probably not the best for most patient education programs. Instead, write objectives about what you want the patients to accomplish by lowering cholesterol or blood pressure, stopping smoking, taking medications as directed, following an exercise program, etc. If the outcome does not make a difference, then it probably should not be included as an objective. Rereading the first part of this chapter on choosing content should help you in forming your objectives.

❑ CRITERIA FOR THE ACTION

This part of the objective answers the questions who, what, when, where, for example, 'after the course', 'the participants', 'the siblings of burn patients', 'cholesterol or blood pressure reading', 'given a choice of cooking oils'. If you do not know who is going to do something, and how, when, or where they are going to do it, then there is no way of judging if it happens.

❑ CRITERIA FOR JUDGING IF THE ACTION HAPPENS

This part of the objective answers the question of how many or how much. It almost always deals with numbers. For example, 8% of the participants, diastolic blood pressure of 90 or below, increase at least ten points, four blocks, three times a week. Without these criteria you have no way of knowing if you reached your objective. It is fine to say that patients will lower their blood pressure. However, you also need to know how many participants lower their blood pressure and by how much. Is a program successful if two out of 100 patients accomplish what you want them to accomplish? Probably not.

Having examined how to write objectives, let us now look at how these can be applied to program planning. First, you should write only a few (less than ten) overall objectives for your program. These program objectives also form the basis for your outcome evaluation. See page 16. Then write objectives for each session or patient encounter. For example, the overall objective for a hypertension course might be: at the end of the course, 70% of the participants will have a diastolic pressure below 90. The objectives for session one of a hypertension course might be:

Participants will:

1   discuss three ways of lowering blood pressure

2   choose one behavior they will change in the coming week

In addition, process objectives should be written. These can usually be standardized for the entire intervention and do not need to be written for each session. Examples of these are:

Instructors will:

1   take attendance at every class

2   ensure that all participants say something at every session

3   reinforce verbally or nonverbally (with nods of head, etc.) every person in every class

4   ensure that 80% of the participants make a commitment to some activity at the end of sessions 2-6

5   use brainstorming as a problem solving technique

These process objectives form the basis for your process evaluation. See page 16.

In summary, objectives tell you where you are going and how you are going to get there. Writing them may seem burdensome. However, the very process of writing process and outcome objectives forces you to clarify your thinking. More importantly, writing objectives enables you to communicate what you are thinking to others. Finally, objectives give you standards by which to evaluate your program.

Process

By now you have chosen your content and written your objectives. The next step is to plan your process or how you are going to teach. In achieving behavior change and changes in health status, process is at least as important as content and probably more important. As a general rule of thumb, it is a good idea to use several different processes each session. Also, the more interactive and participatory, the more likely change will occur. In this section, let's discuss a number of commonly used methods for teaching patient education.

National Mass Media

Mass media can take many forms, each with its own advantages and disadvantages. For example, newspaper, radio, and TV can reach large numbers of people and are excellent for making the public aware of a single need or event. It would not make much sense to use a small group or even a lecture format to try to inform people about an impending flood. On the other hand, mass media are very expensive unless you use free public service announcements. The problem with free media is that you have no control over when your message will be released or sometimes the exact content of the message. To get good free use of the media requires a lot of press cultivation. Mass media, unless there is a huge amount and the message is very simple, is not good at changing health behaviors. Remember, stopping smoking is much more complicated than changing brands of detergent.

Local Media

Local media are an often overlooked form of media which, in most communities, is free for public access. While it is true that local stations sometimes do not have a big audience, they can be used in some creative ways. For example, the Stanford Heart Disease Prevention Project produced a group of smoking cessation programs. The programs used a lecture/discussion format with a local media personality going through the program on TV. People were urged to watch individually or in small groups. There was a great deal of advance publicity to let people know about the coming programs. However, this was still a targeted audience of several thousand people. Of course in using local media, production time and skills are fairly complex. Nevertheless, these can often be donated by students and others. A final advantage to the use of local media is that, if skilfully done, it can combine the advantages of mass media and small group.

Computer-Based Education (CBE)

Computers are now becoming widely available in schools, libraries and some homes. They are a much underutilized medium for health education. The advantage of computer-based education (CBE) is that it can reach a large audience. For example, there are programs on stress management, weight loss and arthritis. These programs can be placed in schools and workplaces, as well as in health care settings. CBE can be somewhat individually tailored and can be paced to the needs of the individual. Once produced, it is relatively inexpensive. The disadvantage is that good production, as with any health education materials, requires both educational and technical skills. Also, CBE software must have compatible computers on which to run.

Films/Video Tapes

These are excellent if you know exactly why you are using any one particular film. Movies or videos allow you to illustrate something, sometimes in a more entertaining way, than you could in an ordinary educational setting. In addition, they can illustrate some skills which are more difficult to show in a class setting, such as exercise or food preparation. If patients have VCRs, video tapes can be taken home to reinforce new behaviors. This is especially true for exercise programs. Finally, video tapes may be a means of providing education for patients with relatively rare diseases.

The disadvantage is that the film may not be exactly what you want to say, and thus may give a false impression, or the video may have little to do with the lives of the audience. Showing a Dairy Council film with

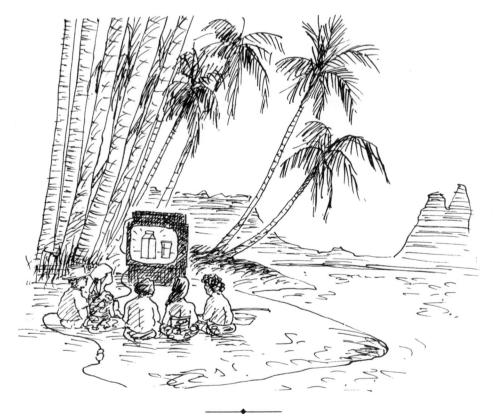

emphasis on milk products and European eating habits to South Pacific islanders does not make much sense. Inner city teenagers may have a hard time relating to films on baby sitting which feature suburban life. The classic example of the problem with films was a cartoon film developed for Third World countries on how flies spread disease. The message was clear and the film entertaining. The only problem was that most people did not feel it applied to their situation because they did not have flies as large as those in the cartoon.

One last drawback to films and tapes is that they take equipment which may or may not work and may or may not be fixable. To be safe, any time you plan to use film or other media which require equipment, be prepared to continue your program without it.

Combined Media Programs

Many people live in rural or semi-rural environments. Therefore, many of the methods mentioned are difficult and just not cost-effective. The result is that large segments of the population are denied programs. The simplest and most often used solution to this problem is the use of printed materials. There have been several programs which have combined media sources bringing some of the advantages of small groups into rural areas. The Utah Lung Association developed an audio tape and booklet program on chronic obstructive pulmonary disease which they sent to clients in rural areas. After people had used the tapes, they were visited by a Lung Association representative who answered questions.

The University of Virginia has developed a rural arthritis program. Each week or two participants are sent an audio tape and booklet. The participants read the booklet, listen to the tape, fill out worksheets and then return the sheets to the university along with their questions. These are answered by phone or in writing and the next lesson is sent. In this way, one person in a centralized location can cover hundreds of miles. Both of these programs have resulted in improvement in health status for their participants.

Having examined some media-centered processes, let us now examine some of the processes useful in one to one and small group education.

Brainstorming

This is one of the most common ways of gaining group participation in a non-threatening manner. In addition to gaining participation, brainstorming is useful for creating many ideas and/or forming new ideas. Although it is often used, brainstorming is at times done incorrectly. Proper brainstorming consists of five steps.

❑ First, participants are given directions. For example, 'I will ask you a question and then you should give as many ideas as you can. Don't worry if the ideas sound silly or are a little strange. If you don't understand what someone else says, don't worry; we will talk about this later. Right now, all I want is for you to give as many ideas as you can.'

❑ Second, ask the question. It is important that the question be properly asked. To do this, it is best to write out the question before you begin your teaching. Don't say, 'Give me some ideas about problems with medications'; rather, say 'What are some of the reasons why people do not take medications as prescribed by their doctor?' The first question is too vague and will result in all kinds of strange answers while the second question is geared specifically to finding out why people do not comply with medication regimens.

❑ Third, write down whatever the members of the group say. Keep writing items until no more are generated. Do not stop to discuss items. Just clarify that you are writing down what the participants say. It is useful to have two people conducting a brainstorm. One monitors the group for responses while the other writes. If you are the only trainer, you might ask someone in the group to write for you. However, be sure that the person writes what is actually said, not his or her interpretation.

❑ Fourth, ask if anyone needs clarification on what any of the items means. Have the person originally offering the item give the clarification.

❑ Fifth and finally, once all the items have been clarified, you can use the brainstorm material to summarize a point, begin a problem solving session or as a point of departure for further teaching or discussion. For example, you want to emphasize the advantages of exercise. Instead of giving a lecture, have the participants brainstorm all the advantages. Then you can correct any misconceptions or add the one or two things the group forgot. Another use of brainstorms is to problem-solve. Someone in the group has a problem, such as not being able to avoid all the tempting food brought to work by coworkers. Instead of the leader offering solutions, ask the group for solutions. Then have the person with the problem indicate the one or two solutions he will try.

Role Playing

There are at least two reasons why role playing might be used in patient education. First, it allows participants to discuss issues which they might otherwise feel were too sensitive. More often, role playing is used to help participants practice a new skill or to rehearse for a future difficult situation. It should be noted that role playing is a difficult training skill and should only be used by a patient educator who is comfortable with the technique. Also, participants often feel threatened and therefore do not like to role-play. No one likes to be on display, especially if they might be made to look foolish. There are several variations of role playing which help to control the situation and protect the participants.

COACHING

Give the participants a situation. For example, pretend that you are expressing dissatisfaction to your doctor. One person plays the doctor and one the patient. After the patient has expressed dissatisfaction, make some suggestion of how he or she might have done this differently, and then reenact the role play using your alternative. A variation on this is to ask members of the group for suggestions on how they might change the interaction. Again, it is important that the 'patient' practice whatever solution is chosen. A second variation is to role-play in threes. One person is the doctor, the second the patient, the third the coach. In this case, have three situations, so that everyone has a chance to play each role.

TRAINER PARTICIPATION

In this situation, the patient educator takes one of the roles. For example, if a participant expresses difficulty in communicating with her child, the trainer would take the role of the child. In this way the trainer can be sure that the responses are not too off the wall or threatening to the participant.

GROUP ROLE PLAYS

Here the trainer plays one role, for example, a patient who is very concerned about surgery, and the whole group plays the second role, for example, the nurse. First, one person counsels the 'patient' and if he or she gets stuck then someone else in the group takes over. This is a very non-threatening form of role playing and is easily controlled by the trainer.

Rehearsal

This is one of the most useful forms of role play. Give the patient a situation which she might encounter. For example, a post cardiac patient on a low calorie diet goes out to eat with friends who urge her to have dessert. The patient can then practice refusal skills. People who rehearse difficult situations before actually encountering them do better when faced with them in the real world. By the way, rehearsal can easily be combined with coaching or group role plays.

Questioning

This is one of the most important of all patient education skills. Not only does it enable you to find out what the patient knows but can also be a useful way of teaching new skills. A very basic rule for all questioning is that you should very seldom ask questions which can be answered by a 'yes' or 'no'. Open-ended questions are much better. Do not ask, 'Are you feeling better today?' Ask, 'How are you feeling today?'

The following are some ways you might use questioning in your patient teaching:

❏ *The patient knows what he or she should do but is not doing it.*

Ask, 'Why do you smoke?' 'What are you afraid might happen if you lost weight?' 'What problems do you think you might have in starting an exercise program?'

❏ *You are helping a patient solve a problem.*

Ask, 'What solutions do you see for this problem?' 'Where might you go to get other ideas?' 'Which of these solutions would you like to try?' It is always better to teach problem solving skills than to solve problems. Of course, in some situations, it is best to give an answer. If a patient asks which type of oil is low in cholesterol, there is no reason to cause frustration by telling him to go to the library.

One note of caution about questioning. Keep your voice tone neutral. Sometimes, when poorly asked, questions become judgmental. For example, 'Why do *you* smoke?' instead of, '*Why* do you smoke?'.

Self-Monitoring

One of the best ways to get people to change behaviors is to let them monitor their own experience. People have a difficult time denying their own evidence. On the more positive side, self-monitoring helps a person see his or her problems or progress. Examples of self-monitoring include keeping a food diary or keeping track of when headaches occur. This information can then be used as the basis for behavior change. Self-monitoring can also be used as feedback, such as weekly weigh-ins and keeping track of exercise progress. This is like the feedback which is so important for obtaining skills mastery. For more on self-monitoring and skills mastery, see page 111.

Creative patient educators can almost always build some self-monitoring techniques into their programs. The following are more concrete examples.

A DIET
In many cases we are trying to change our diet. This may be to lose weight, to lower cholesterol, to increase calcium, to decrease fats, or to conform to some regimen such as a diabetic diet. In all these cases, a good place to start is to have the patient keep a four-day diet history in which he writes down everything he eats as he eats it. The four days should probably be two weekend days and two weekdays. Fridays are more like weekend days than weekdays and thus should probably not be counted in the four days. This self-monitoring of food intake helps him to see where the problems lie and make plans to change. After being on a program for a while, he can again do a four-day diary to see progress and check for any new problems.

B EXERCISE
There are several ways to monitor exercise. The time spent exercising, the distance covered, the weights lifted, or the number of repetitions all serve to help people see how they are progressing. While exercising, she can take her own pulse to be sure that she is in an aerobic zone. A quick self-monitoring test is that if she cannot talk while exercising, unless of course she is swimming, then she is exercising too much. Such simple self-monitoring guidelines are helpful in getting people started.

C   DIABETES
Urine testing and blood glucose monitoring are both good ways of helping a diabetic self-monitor.

D   HYPERTENSION
We know that many people have white coat hypertension. That is, their blood pressure is much higher in the doctor's office than at any other time. Therefore, self-monitoring is very helpful. This can be done by getting the client to have his blood pressure taken regularly. This might be done at senior centers, at the blood bank when giving blood, or at special health awareness weeks like National Health Week. You might even teach clients how to take their own blood pressures and have equipment available at a convenient location. It is not important that the readings be 100% accurate. Rather, the client can see how his blood pressure changes over time. Of course, he needs a little instruction in the meaning of the numbers.

E   WEIGHT LOSS
Scales are wonderful self-monitoring devices.

F   ASTHMA
Here you are trying to teach symptom recognition as well as to get people to act on their symptoms before they become serious. Monitoring can include keeping track of the number of times she must call the doctor, go into emergency, or miss work because of asthma. Also, she can keep track of when medication is taken and its relationship to the seriousness of the attack. Peak flow meters are also excellent.

There are no doubt hundreds of other ways to help people self-monitor. The more of these that you can build into the program, the more chance you will have of seeing real behavior change.

Having examined several teaching methods, let's now turn to determining who is going to teach. It is usually best to decide who is going to present your program before it is developed. In this way you can include the presenters in program development. No one likes to be told to do something when they have had no input. However, sometimes, the program presenters are chosen only after the program is fully developed.

This is especially true with very standardized programs.

One to One Education

This is the most common type of patient education. It is what doctors, nurses and other health professionals do at the bedside or in the clinic. In one to one education there are four major considerations: time, knowing what to teach, knowing how to teach, and documenting what has been taught.

Time is an especially valuable commodity for doctors and, to a slightly less extent, for other health care professionals. Most doctors have only ten to twenty minutes in which to interact with a patient. Therefore, any education must be very quick. Some have called these thirty-second interventions. So what can you do in thirty seconds? Heaps. A doctor can tell a patient, 'I want you to stop smoking.' This is one of the most powerful things a doctor can do to get someone to stop smoking. When doing a breast examination, the doctor can ask the patient to demonstrate how she examines her breasts. It has been found that getting a woman to touch her own breast is one of the best ways of assuring future breast self-examination. Patients receiving prescriptions should always be asked how they are going to take the medication. This simple question helps to reveal any problems or misunderstandings. For example, one patient I know, when given an antibiotic labeled 'Avoid exposure to sunlight', was very careful to keep the pills in a dark place. She never considered that she should avoid exposure to sun. Finally, the doctor can make referrals. 'I know that you want to lose weight; here is a list of resources in our community to help you with that effort.' The above examples are just a few of the many possible thirty-second interventions. In planning what you want doctors to do, it is important to be realistic.

Nurses, physical therapists, occupational therapists and other health professionals also have limited time. However, it may not be as limited as that of a doctor. Therefore, you might think of three- to five-minute interventions which can realistically take place in the context of normal practice. By using some of the priority setting techniques discussed on page 31, these few minutes can be well utilized. In all cases it is important to separate out what a patient wants and needs to know from what the health professional wants to teach. The priority should always be on the first two.

Knowing What to Teach

Unfortunately, very few health professionals when working with patients one to one give much thought as to what they should teach. There is just not time. Therefore, it is important that this decision process occur before the actual patient encounter. Thus, if a patient is in for bypass surgery, there should be a set protocol of things to teach. In fact, a checklist can be made up and then checked off as the patient education is delivered. The problem is not that professionals don't know the content. It is usually that they know too much and try to teach it all. Or they decide wisely that it is impossible to teach it all and therefore decide to teach nothing. In neither case are patient needs served. Again, what is needed is a priority setting process which clarifies for all professionals what they should be teaching to any specific patient.

Knowing How to Teach

Now this is the big one. Most health professionals believe that they know how to teach. The reality is that most of them are only poor to fair patient educators. There are several reasons for this. First, few have had any formal training in patient education. Lacking this training, they try to emulate the teaching that they have received. The problem with this approach is that most school-type teaching is aimed at passing on knowledge. Patient education is aimed at changing behaviors or health status. Thus, the teaching methods are different and must be learned and practiced.

In planning patient education programs it is often necessary to teach patient education skills to the patient-educators. These skills include the use of questioning, problem solving, goal setting, as well as demonstration and return demonstration. All of these are discussed elsewhere (pages 43, 111, 114). The important thing to note is that sometimes preparing a program is not enough. Significant time and effort must be spent on preparing health professionals to take on the role of successful patient educators.

Documenting What You Teach

There are at least two major reasons for documenting what you teach. First, in many places, this is a requirement for hospital accreditation. More important, for programs to be successful, it is necessary to know what patients have been taught and what they still need to learn. In this way, a patient won't be taught about hypertension medications five times and never learn the importance of exercise.

Documentation can take many forms. If there is a set protocol, let us say a six session diabetes course, then all you need to do is to document that a patient attended the course and that the protocol was delivered as written. Unfortunately, documentation is not always this easy. In one to one teaching, it is helpful to note in the chart what has been taught. The problem is that few people will go back through pages of chart notes to figure out what to teach next. Charting may be helpful for legal purposes but may not help the patient.

An alternative is to have a patient education page in the chart. This is easy to find and also serves as documentation. The disadvantage is that it adds bulk to the chart. A variation of the patient education chart is to have a checklist of all the things that a patient should be taught about any set condition. Then, when something is taught, the item can be checked off and initialed. This is even more effective if the checklist is kept on the patient's bed. In this case anyone who does any education —nurses, physical therapists, occupational therapists and doctors—can see what has already been done and what is left to do. This checklist can then be placed in the permanent chart when the patient goes home. Similar types of checklists can be kept in outpatient charts. In all cases it is important to be clear on how the documentation will be used. There is no reason to go to all this trouble if the documentation has no meaning

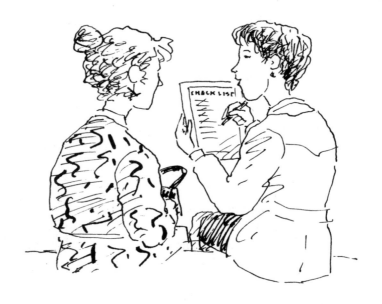

for the patient, for program planning or as a legal document.

Group Education

Everything that we have said about one to one education is also true for group education. The difference is that the patient educator must have a greater variety of skills. In addition to all the one to one skills mentioned above, the educator, if he or she is going to do more than just lecture, must have skills in group process. Again, you are not born with these skills but rather learn them from life experience or in a structured manner. A complete program for training patient educators is beyond the scope of this book. However, it is important to be aware of the possibility that you may need to train your patient educators or to see that they receive training. Like everything else, patient education process is learned. It is not inherited.

Putting It All Together

So far we have looked at many of the pieces which are necessary for putting together a patient education program. However, the real trick of patient education is putting the content and process together in a package which helps patients to reach the outcome objectives. Such packaging usually takes the form of a protocol, which outlines the general topics to be covered in the program. Good patient education protocols should also be so detailed that someone who is not familiar with the program can pick it up and replicate what you are doing. The reason such detailed protocols are not usually done is that they require a lot of thought and preparation.

In preparing a protocol there are several things to keep in mind. First, write your objectives and be sure that what you are teaching is designed to meet these objectives. For example, if you want a cardiac patient to exercise, do not spend the majority of your time on explaining disease process. If you want an intervention to be interactive, use as little lecture as possible and build in interactive activities. These do not just happen; they have to be planned.

Second, make sure that you vary your activities. Everyone gets tired of the same format. Thus, you might include some lecture, brainstorming, a film, and general discussion, all in one session. It is especially important to encourage active participation of group members after lunch or dinner as these are times that people sometimes get sluggish or are apt to fall asleep. A good time to introduce new activities is early in the day when people are fresh. Another trick of the trade is to save some of your most interesting material until last. This encourages people to stay to the end instead of leaving early.

Third, if at all possible, build on activities over several weeks. Thus, rather than having one session on diet and another on exercise, have two or more sessions which include and/or add to both of these subjects. In this way participants will have a chance to go home, decide what they want to do, try things out, and report back with problems. Then there is still time to make changes.

Finally, try to use the same instructors or facilitator for every session. This builds in continuity and helps to create rapport between the instructors and participants, which is especially important for group education. If you use a different 'expert' every session this is not patient education; it is a lecture series. While there is nothing wrong with a lecture series, it is important to understand that it is very unlikely that such a series will result in behavior change. However, lecture series are usually very good for increasing knowledge.

The following is the protocol from the first two-hour session of the Arthritis Self-Help course (Lorig). This patient education program is offered by the Arthritis Foundations of the United States and Australia and by the Arthritis Societies in Canada. The course is designed to be taught by a pair of leaders, at least one of whom is a lay person with arthritis. Self-efficacy theory serves as the theoretical framework for the course. As you read over this protocol, note that the session has specific objectives and the activities are varied, starting with an interactive exercise.

Activity 1 sets the tone for the following 12 hours. It clearly sets forth the expectations for the group's participation by reviewing the 'rules' (chart 2). Also, within the first few minutes, there is a course overview (chart 3) which helps participants decide if they have come to the right course.

Activity 2 reinforces this tone during a brief lecturette on self-help principles.

Activity 3 is an example of helping participants to reinterpret physiological signs and symptoms. This is one of the ways to enhance self-efficacy (page 109). Note that this activity again is done in an interactive mode rather than lecture.

Activity 4 is a lecture on the disease process. These 15 minutes are the only ones during 12 hours of education devoted to disease process. Chart 4, as well as the other charts, is used to reinforce information which is given through lecture or other means.

Activity 5 is the first introduction to exercise. This topic is repeated and built upon during each of the following five sessions. Note that this activity uses both brainstorming and lecture.

Activity 6 is the ending for every class. Contracting is used to assist participants in gaining skills mastery. This is another important component for building self-efficacy. Note that this activity ends with a short visualization exercise to help participants fix their contract in their minds, as well as their success in accomplishing the contract.

In summary, this two-hour session has used several educational processes including the group's sharing of experience, lecturette, visual charts, brainstorming, a short self-quiz, contracting, and visualization. In addition, it has covered several content areas including a needs assessment, discussion of disease process, and introduction to exercise. In short, this first session sets the stage for the use of content and process for the entire 12 hours.

Session One

Purpose:
❑   To introduce the group members to each other
❑   To inform the group about the general principles of self-help
❑   To identify the group members' feelings about arthritis
❑   To provide basic information about arthritis
❑   To introduce group members to the importance of exercise

Objectives:
By the end of this session, the group members will be able to:
1   state their role in the care of their arthritis.
2   define the differences between the major types of arthritis.
3   state the benefits of physical fitness for arthritis.
4   state the 3 parts of an exercise program.
5   make a contract for an arthritis-related behavior in the coming week.

Materials:
❑ Blank name tags for everyone
❑ Easel
❑ Blank flip charts/felt pens or blackboard chalk, pre-written Charts 1-5
❑ *The Arthritis Helpbook* for each person
❑ Pad of paper, extra pencils

Plan Outline *(Post this agenda at the beginning of class)*:
Activity 1 Introduction (25 min)
        2 Overview of Self-Help Principles (10 min)
        3 Debunking Myths (10 min)
Break (10 min)
Activity 4 Introduction to Arthritis (15 min)
        5 Exercising: Start Where You Are (20 min)
        6 Contracting (20 min)
        7 Closing (5 min)

Activity 1: INTRODUCTION (25 min)

Methods: Lecturette and group introductions
Note: Refer to Charts 1-3

Charts are shown throughout this manual with the material to be printed on the chart in bold caps (and the material you add verbally bracketed).

1 As participants arrive, distribute name tags. Have them write the names they like to be called—large enough so that they can be read across the room. Also, collect physician information forms (if necessary).

2 Welcome the group and introduce yourself, including the fact that you have arthritis (if true).

3 Group introductions. Have participants write down what arthritis means to them. Then have participants introduce themselves and share what arthritis means to them. One leader should list what people say on the board or chart pad (Chart 1). Put a check mark next to a word or statement every time it is repeated by another person.

Chart 1
WHAT ARTHRITIS MEANS TO ME

Note: Save this chart (*Chart 1* - WHAT ARTHRITIS MEANS TO ME) to make comparisons of progress in the last session.

4   Describe the 'rules' of the group. Refer to Chart 2.

Chart 2
'RULES'

1   **COME TO EVERY SESSION.**

2   **ASK ANYTHING YOU WANT.** (If we don't know the answer, we will get it. Also, if time is short, we may ask you to hold your questions for later.)

3   **DO YOUR HOMEWORK.** (It won't be graded but will make the course more valuable to you.)

4   **GIVE NEW ACTIVITIES AT LEAST A TWO-WEEK TRIAL** (before deciding what will work best for you.)

5   **MAKE AND COMPLETE A WEEKLY CONTRACT.**

---

5   Using Chart 3, give an overview of the course. Comment on how the content relates to 'what arthritis means' to group members by referring back to their statements made at the beginning of the session (which you have on Chart 1).

Chart 3
COURSE OVERVIEW

Session 1:   **Self-Help Principles**
                  Myths
                  Disease Process (OA/RA)
                  Exercise/Fitness
                  Feedback/Contracting

Session 2:   **Flexibility/Strengthening Exercise**
                  Pain Management/Relaxation
                  Feedback/Contracting

Session 3:   **Aerobic Exercise**
                  Depression

> **Distraction**
> **Guided Imagery**
> **Feedback/Contracting**
>
> *Session 4:* **Nutrition**
> **Osteoporosis**
> **Non-Traditional Treatments**
> **Self-Talk**
> **Problem-Solving**
> **Feedback/Contracting**
>
> *Session 5:* **Communication Skills**
> **Working With Your Doctor**
> **Fitness Progress**
> **Visualization**
> **Feedback/Contracting**
>
> *Session 6:* **Medications**
> **Fatigue**
> **Sharing Accomplishments**
> **Feedback/Contracting - Future Goals**

6   If participants show an interest in topics that will not be addressed (such as surgery or research), state that they can probably find that information in *The Arthritis Helpbook*. If not, they can call the local Arthritis Foundation/Society.

Activity 2:   OVERVIEW OF SELF-HELP PRINCIPLES (10 min)
Introduction to the participative nature of this course

Method: Lecturette

1   Although the cure for arthritis is unknown, there are a variety of known treatments to *control* arthritis, i.e. to relieve discomfort and reduce disability. It is your responsibility to learn as much as possible about these treatments.

2   Self-help means being willing to learn about and assume responsibility for the daily care of your arthritis.

your arthritis care.

4   Being responsible for your arthritis includes:

   a   Keeping informed about your status—asking questions.

   b   Taking part in planning the treatment program—telling the health care team about your preferences and goals.

   c   Trying out different treatments (under the guidance of your health care team) until you come up with the best treatment program for you.

   d   Setting goals and working toward them.

   e   Informing the health care team about problems and changes you make in your daily program.

Activity 3:   DEBUNKING MYTHS (10 min)

Methods: Lecturette/Quiz

1   As we pointed out in our preview of the course content, we will be learning and using different strategies to manage our arthritis. Before we begin exploring these, however, we'd like you to answer some questions which reflect some beliefs about arthritis.

2   Ask participants to write whether or not they agree, partially agree or disagree with the following statements about arthritis. Tell them their answers will *not* be collected. Do not take more than a few minutes to complete this exercise.

   Read the following:

   a   If you are feeling tired or fatigued, you should always rest.

   b   If exercise hurts, you shouldn't exercise.

   c   The best diet for someone with arthritis is one low in fats and high in fiber.

   d   One can easily injure joints by exercising.

e   Arthritis pain is caused mainly by damaged joints.

f   Health professionals are the best people to solve arthritis
    problems.

3   After the group has finished writing their responses, cover the
    following explanations. Note that these are based on what we now
    know from the latest arthritis research. Mention again that these
    topics will be discussed more completely in later sessions, referring
    to Chart 3. Responses:

a   While fatigue is a symptom of the disease process, feeling tired
    can also be caused by stress or other emotions. Therefore, many
    people may find that exercise actually gives them more energy
    and that rest is not always appropriate.

b   Many times people confuse arthritis pain with exercise-induced
    pain caused by weak or sore muscles. We will talk more about the
    difference between these in the next class and provide some
    guidelines for telling them apart. Exercising will actually help
    lessen the pain when done correctly, but if you allow the pain to
    stop you from ever starting you won't get anywhere. The bottom
    line is that if you can move, you can exercise.

c   A diet low in fats and high in fiber is desirable for good health,
    in general. Diets recommended by the Heart Foundation and the
    American Cancer Society are good ones to follow. There is no
    specific 'arthritis' diet.

d   It is very difficult to cause permanent damage to joints by
    exercising. In fact, by using the proper exercise techniques, the
    joint is strengthened and supported better, not damaged. Exer-
    cises like walking, swimming and bicycling can all help arthritis
    and contribute to overall improved fitness.

e   Some arthritis pain is caused by damaged joints. However, much
    of arthritis pain is also caused by stress, tight or weak muscles
    and emotions. In this course we will learn ways to deal with all
    kinds of arthritis pain.

f   Only you can solve your problems. Health professionals, family and friends can all make suggestions. However, only you make the final decisions about what to do and how to carry out your program. You are in charge!

BREAK (10 min)

Activity 4: INTRODUCTION TO ARTHRITIS (15 min)

Background Reading: *Helpbook,* pp. 1-16.
Methods: Lecturette/Discussion
Note: Refer to picture of joint on p. 2 of *Helpbook.*

1. Classic definition of 'arthritis' — diseases of joints.

2. If anything goes wrong with any part of the joint, it is usually arthritis.

3. Now known to be not one disease but more than 100 different diseases.

4. No known cure for most forms of arthritis, therefore self-management of symptoms is important.

5. Anatomy of joint: bone, muscle, cartilage, tendon, bursa, and synovial membrane (see *Helpbook*, p. 2).

6. Difference between osteoarthritis (OA) and rheumatoid arthritis (RA). Have participants refer to the *Helpbook*, p. 3.

Types of Arthritis

	OSTEOARTHRITIS	RHEUMATOID ARTHRITIS
Pathology: What happens	Cartilage degeneration; bone regeneration (spurs).	Inflammation of synovial membrane, bone destruction, damage to ligaments, tendons.
Joints Affected	Hands, spine, knees, hips. May be asymmetrical (one-sided).	Wrists, knees, knuckles; symmetrical (both sides).
Features: Symptoms	Localized pain, stiffness, Heberden's nodules; usually not much swelling.	Swelling, redness, warmth, pain, tenderness, nodules, fatigue, stiffness, muscle aches, fever.
Prognosis:	Less pain for some, more pain and	Less aggressive with time; deformity

Long-term	disability for others. Few severely disabled.	can often be prevented.
Age: Onset	Age 45-90. Most of us have some features with increasing age.	Adults aged 20–50.
Sex: Heredity	Males and females equally. The form with knobby fingers runs in families.	75% female, 1/2 of 1% of US population. Familial tendency.
Tests	X-rays	Rheumatoid factor (80%), blood tests, x-rays, examination of joint fluid.
Treatment	Maintain activity level, exercise, joint protection, weight control, relaxation, heat, sometimes medication and/or surgery.	Reduce inflammation, balanced exercise program, joint protection, weight control, relaxation, heat, usually medication, sometimes surgery.

Note: This section is deliberately brief. Encourage participants to read the *Helpbook* this week and bring any questions they have to the next class.

Activity 5: EXERCISE FOR FUN AND FITNESS—WHERE TO START (20 min)

Background Reading: *Helpbook*, pp. 35-47
Methods: Lecturette/Discussion
Note: Refer to Chart 4

1 In this course, we will talk about exercise for fun and fitness. Just because you have arthritis is no reason why you should not be fit and enjoy exercise.

2 Brainstorm: What does it mean to be fit?
After the brainstorm, be sure that these five points are covered:

  1 Strong cardiovascular system—heart and blood vessels

  2 Good strength

  3 Good endurance/stamina

  4 Good flexibility

  5 Low percentage of body fat—proper weight

3 A good fitness program accomplishes all of the above and more. It has 3 parts (refer to Chart 4):

Chart 4
3 PARTS OF A FITNESS PROGRAM

WARM-UP - (for muscle strength and flexibility; preparation for aerobic exercise)

AEROBIC EXERCISE - (for cardiovascular fitness, endurance and weight control)

COOL DOWN - (for body relaxation and to avoid sore muscles)

---

4   A warm-up routine usually consists of some flexibility/strengthening exercises and a gradual increase in aerobic activity. When you are able to do 15 minutes of flexibility/strengthening exercises you are ready to move on to your aerobic activity. Remember to cool down afterwards with a gradual decrease in activity and some more flexibility/strengthening exercise.

5   There are as many fitness programs as there are people. One example is a warm-up which includes slow walking, followed by a few minutes of brisker walking, and then a few more minutes of slow walking again. If you are just beginning a program, start by walking slowly for 3-5 minutes. Build up gradually until you can walk 15 minutes. If you can already walk 15 minutes, start by walking slowly for 5-10 minutes, and then walk briskly for 5-20 minutes, ending with a slow walk to cool down for 5-10 minutes. The basic principle is to start by doing whatever you can do now, 3-4 times a week, and build up from there gradually.

6   During this course, we want each of you to chart your fitness progress. There are very few of us who in some way could not be more fit. For homework this week, ask everyone to think about how they would like to improve their fitness and be ready to report on this next week, as well as on what they can do now.

Activity 6:   CONTRACTING (20 min)

Background Reading: *Helpbook,* pp. 27-33
Methods: Lecturette/Discussion
Note: Refer to Chart 5

1   Over the years, we have found that the self-helpers who accomplish the most are the ones who set short-term goals. Therefore, in this class, we will be asking each of you to make a contract each week for something *you* want to accomplish. For example, a contract might be: 'This week I'll walk 3 blocks before lunch on 4 days,' or 'This week I'll not eat after dinner 4 nights,' or 'This week I'll practice relaxation techniques for 15 minutes 3 nights after dinner.'

2   The rules for making a contract are (refer to Chart 5):

> **Chart 5**
> **RULES OF CONTRACTING**
>
> 1   **IDENTIFY SOMETHING YOU WANT TO DO**
>
> 2   **BE REALISTIC**
>
> 3   **SPECIFY** — what, when, how many or how much
>
> 4   **WRITE IT DOWN**
>
> 5   **CHECK IT DAILY**

3   Leaders give examples of the contracts they will do in the next week.

4   If the group is more than 10, break the class into two groups with one leader in each group.

5   Introduce participants to the contract form in their *Helpbook*, p. 33. Ask participants to write a contract for the week.

6   Have participants read their contracts and tell how confident they are that they can accomplish it (100 is very certain, 0 is not at all certain). Emphasize that this number is *not* the percentage of the contract they believe they can complete, but how certain they are

that they can complete the *whole* contract. If 100 or 90, suggest the contract may be too easy. If 70 or less, suggest the contract may be too hard. In either case, suggest that the participant adjust the contract. (To help people contract, see contracting script.)

7   If someone is having trouble writing a clear contract (i.e. specific activity, times per day, days per week), ask other group members for suggestions *before* you help. Do not spend more than 3-4 minutes with any one person. If someone is having problems, work with them individually *after* class.

8   While still in contracting groups, have participants close their eyes, take 3 deep breaths, and think about themselves successfully fulfilling their contracts. Read Script 1 (when reading the script wait a few seconds every time you see the dots ...) or, if time permits, use the 'visualization to achieve your goals' exercise on the leader's tape.

Script One

Close your eyes...now take 3 deep breaths: in through your nose and out through your mouth...see yourself easily carrying out the activity in your contract...(30-45 seconds of silence)...think about how good you feel...take 3 more deep breaths and open your eyes.

9   Inform the participants that the class leaders will be calling them once during the coming week to support them in their contract.

Contract Script

I   *Deciding what one wants to accomplish*

Ask the person, 'What will you do this week?' It is important that the activity come from the participant and *not* you. This activity does not have to be something covered in class—just something that the participant wants to do to change behavior. Do not let anyone say, 'I will try...' Each person should say, 'I will...'

II   *Making a plan*

This is the difficult and most important part of contracting. Part I is worthless without Part II. The plan should contain all of the following elements:

1 *Exactly what* is the participant going to do (i.e. how far will you walk, how will you eat less, what relaxation techniques will you practice)?

2 *How much* (i.e. walk around the block, 15 minutes, etc.)?

3 *When* will the participant do this? Again, this must be specific (i.e. before lunch, in the shower, when I come home from work).

4 *How often* will the activity be done? This is a bit tricky. Most participants tend to say every day. In contracting, the most important thing is to succeed. Therefore, it is better to contract to do something 4 times a week and exceed the contract by actually doing it 5 times than to contract to do something every day and fail by only doing it 6 days. To ensure success, we usually encourage people to contract to do something 3 to 5 days a week. Remember that success and self-efficacy are as important, or maybe even more important, than actually doing the behavior.

III *Checking the contract*

Once the contract is complete, ask the participant 'Given a scale of 0 to 100, with 0 being totally unsure and 100 being totally certain, how certain are you that you will (repeat the participant's contract verbatim)?'

If the answer is 70 or above, this is probably a realistic contract and the participant should write it on his or her contract sheet.

If the answer is below 70, then the contract should be reassessed. Ask the participant: 'What makes you uncertain? What problems do you foresee?' Then discuss the problems. Ask other participants to offer solutions. *You should offer solutions last.* Once the problem solving is completed, have the participant restate the contract and return to repeat Part III, checking the contract.

Notes: This contracting process may seem cumbersome and time consuming. However, it does work and is well worth the effort. The first time you contract with a group, plan 2-3 minutes per person. Contracting is a learned skill. Your participant will soon be saying 'I will——4 times this week before lunch and am 80% certain I can do this.' Thus, after two or three contracting sessions, contracting should take less than a minute per participant.

Activity 7: CLOSING (5 min)

1   Invite participants to review what was covered today for next week in the *Helpbook*:

>   Chapters 1-3, pp. 1–16
>   Chapter 6, pp. 27–33.

2   Remind participants to keep track of their contracts daily and to bring them to class next week.

3   Remind participants to think about what they will do to gain greater fitness and be ready to report this next week.

4   Ask participants to bring their books to class each week. Also ask them to bring a tape measure or ruler next week.

5   Tell people to wear comfortable clothes in which they can practice exercises, and ask if 2-4 people will bring blankets which can be put on the floor for exercise. Assure people that the exercise will not be strenuous and no one has to do anything they don't want to do.

6   Thank people for coming and tell them that one of the leaders will be calling them during the week to see how things are going.

7   Collect name tags.

8   Stay around for 15 minutes or so to answer questions and straighten the room.

References

1   Mager, R.F.,
    Preparing Instructional Objectives, Belmont, Calif, Fearon Pub.,
    1970.

2   Lorig, K.,
    Arthritis Self-management Leader's Manual, Atlanta, Arthritis
    Foundation, 1984, revised Oct. 1990.

3   Lorig, K., Fries, J.,
    The Arthritis Helpbook, Reading, Mass, Addison-Wesley, 3rd edition
    Oct. 1990.

How Do I Get
People to Come?

Virginia Gonzalez
and
Kate Lorig

MARKETING AND NETWORKING STRATEGIES

Having the best patient education program in the world does no one any good if no one comes. Low attendance can occur for many reasons. You may have created a product no one wants, people may not know about your program, there are factors which inhibit people from coming, or maybe people are actively discouraged from attending. In this chapter, we will examine ways of marketing your program to health professionals, patients, and special populations that are hard to reach. Finally, we will discuss some ways to utilize community resources to enhance your programs.

Marketing to Health Professionals

Probably the strongest potential allies in marketing your program are other health professionals. At best, they can be very helpful. To be successful, you want to be sure that they are, at least, neutral. At worst, other professionals can completely destroy the program. With this in mind, let's start by examining how to get support from doctors and other health professionals. The time to start your marketing is when you plan your program. In an earlier chapter we talked about an interested parties analysis (see page 3); this is a good technique to involve health professionals.

With health professionals it is important not only to get their input but also to let them be partners in the creation of your program. This does not mean endless group meetings. Rather, when you write content that would be of interest to a doctor, have two or three key doctors review it. Have several doctors review the whole program, offer comments and suggest changes. In choosing your reviewers, do not just choose your friends. Rather, look for opinion leaders, those health professionals who are highly respected by their peers. These might be instructors in health professional programs, officers in professional organizations or senior, well-liked doctors. If your community has factions, for example, two hospitals, then choose reviewers from each faction.

Not only do you want health professionals as reviewers, but you also want to give these people ownership of the program. Ask if you can use their names on handouts or in publicity. When you write to other health professionals about the program, see if your reviewers will cosign your letter. A program invented by Howard Doe, Helen Doe, MD, Chief of

Medicine and Robin Doe, Head PT, may be easily introduced as it comes from credible sources.

Anyone who has ever invented anything has come across the dreaded NIH Syndrome, or Not Invented Here Syndrome. You will recognize the symptoms when you hear, 'That may be the way they do it in New Zealand but not here in Australia' or 'Those people in California just don't understand our health system' or 'People here are different.' The quickest way to defuse this situation is to ask the 'locals' to review the program and work with them to make any specific local adaptions. This forces the locals to look carefully at the program, rather than disliking it from afar. The revisions they make are usually very minor and may even help market the program locally. Most important of all, the local professionals now have ownership of the course so NIH becomes IH, that is, Invented Here.

A second problem we often hear about is, 'We can't get doctors and other health professionals to refer people to our programs.' If you survive the NIH Syndrome, then the problem is probably that your professionals either forget or find making a referral too complicated. Today, most health professionals are very busy. They have very little time and must prioritize what they tell patients. Most do not have adequate time to provide a diagnosis and treatment. Therefore patient education is not in the forefront of their minds. You may not be able to change this but there are a couple of tricks you might try.

Place a poster about your program in the doctor's waiting room or examining room. Have patients tear off tags with the phone number for more information. This way the doctor does not have to do anything, yet the patient understands that the doctor approves of the program. In addition, the poster acts as a stimulus for the patient to ask the doctor for more information or reminds the doctor about the program.

A second method of enlisting help with recruitment from doctors and other health professionals is to place a brightly colored sign-up sheet in the waiting room. The front of the sheet should say something like, 'I am interested in learning more about diabetes education' with spaces for name, address and phone number. The other side of the sheet is preaddressed. Every two weeks or when the sheet is full, whichever occurs first, the office receptionist takes down the sheet and mails it to you. In turn, he or she gets a new sheet. This takes all the responsibility away from the doctor and gets you the information you need.

Another method of getting doctor referrals is to make up special prescription pads (copy shops can do this inexpensively). The doctor then prescribes patient education in much the same way he or she would prescribe a medication.

Sometimes doctors fear that the education program will somehow interfere with their treatment or chase patients away into the hands of another practitioner. To overcome this fear, first assure the doctors that you will always refer their patients back to them. And be sure to do so. Secondly, you might offer to hold the program after hours in the doctor's waiting room. This solves your space problem and assures that a specific doctor is associated with that session of the program.

Within your program, and in your dealings with the public, be very sure to teach that the doctor is not the enemy. Too often, there is a subtle or not so subtle implication that the patient must be on the defensive with doctors. Avoid this at all costs. Secondly, do not play favorites. Even though you may like one doctor better than another, *always* support the patient's choice of doctor. If there are medical questions, suggest that the patient ask his or her doctor. If a patient is unhappy with the doctor, urge a patient-doctor discussion. A doctor once said that doctors will get off their pedestals when patients get off their knees. Our job is to help patients stand, not to knock doctors off their pedestals.

Marketing to the Public

Making Your Program Attractive

Much of the problem in recruiting patients is that your program is not attractive. Some of the common problems are name, cost, time and place.

The title of your program is very important. Self-help for the elderly forces them to admit they are old before enrolling. Growing younger and healthier might be a better title. Hypertension is a symptomless disease, so there may be little motivation on the part of many patients to attend a program. On the other hand, chronic obstructive pulmonary disease (COPD) has painful symptoms; therefore, it might be easier to recruit for COPD Better Breathers programs. Sometimes programs with more than one focus can help. Since a large percentage of older people have arthritis, you might reach more elderly hypertensives with an arthritis/high blood pressure program than with just a high blood pressure program. One way to choose a name, while also resolving some of the other issues discussed in this section, is by using focus groups. You will find details about these on page 9.

Some final hints about naming programs:

❑ Do not be too 'cute'. Illness is a serious matter, especially to the ill. Treating it frivolously often causes anger.

❑ Keep your name simple. No one wants to deal with a fourteen-word name.

❑ Make the name descriptive. The name is what initially attracts people. Asthma Self-Management, Avoiding Heart Attacks, How to Talk With Your Doctor, and Preparing for Labor are all good clear descriptive titles.

Costs

There is a widely held belief among health professionals and others that if someone pays for something they value it more. While this may be true, we have little evidence to suggest that payment makes much difference in terms of behavior change or health status outcome. In fact, if payment were directly linked to outcome, the United States would have the healthiest population in the world! The point here is that you do not have to charge money to make patients appreciate your program. On the other hand, payment may influence attendance or commitment. For example, some weight loss programs charge a high fee and then offer rebates for prespecified weight loss and weight loss maintenance.

You may need to charge to cover the expenses of the program. Usually, the lower or more minimal the fee, the better. This makes your program accessible to everyone. If you must charge more than a minimal fee, you might try a self-policing fee scale. Your application can state that the program costs $25, but that considerations will be made for those with a limited income. Then, as part of the application, have participants check one of the following:

Enclosed is $25.00

I can only afford $———.

Please consider me for a fee waiver

If the fee is reasonable, the public does not take advantage of this offer. In my experience with an arthritis patient education program (the Arthritis Self-Help Course), most people pay the full fee and very few request a complete scholarship. When we charge $10.00, less than 5% of over 1000 patients have asked for a fee waiver. All the rest have paid $10.00. We do not offer the middle option. Often some of the course expenses can be paid for from other sources. For more information about this, see use of community resources on page 78.

Time

It seems obvious that you should hold your program at a convenient time for the clients. Saturday may be a sports day for you but a very lonely day for the elderly. Also, take a look at your competition. Do not hold your hypertension program during the Olympics or on church bingo night. However, it might be successful to hold it at the bingo hall a half hour before bingo. You may even consider offering more than one program on different days, at different times, in order to reach more people.

Place

People are funny. Some places are all right to go and others are not. This has nothing to do with safety. If you want to reach an ethnic population, you might have more success holding the program in a community setting, rather than the hospital. Some Catholics may not go to a Protestant church for a program or vice versa, while others will. Also, some people may cross town for a program but not cross the railroad tracks. People have a range and your program must be given within the range of your audience. Your task is to find out what those ranges are, perhaps through your needs assessment or in a focus group.

Of course, sites must be safe and accessible. Things to consider are stairs, impediments to the physically challenged, parking, public transportation, walking distance, lighting, comfort of chairs, accessibility of toilets and facilities for making coffee and tea. If you are teaching wellness or prevention, hospitals may not be the best places because, in people's minds, that is where sick people go. Hospitals have a negative image for some people. They are also full of 'strange, frightening things', and peculiar smells. For this reason, try to hold your course on neutral ground. Shopping malls, senior centers, hotels, town halls and libraries usually meet this criterion. They are accessible and acceptable to a wide spectrum of the population (see page 79).

Using the Media

So you have done everything right and still no one comes. It may be that no one knows about your program. Good advertising is done in a number of ways. The local media, radio and newspapers, are excellent but also unpredictable if you rely solely on public service announcements. The problem is that you never know when your announcement will get published or be announced. Unfortunately, paid advertising is very expensive. However, for something really important, this may be the way to go.

Sometimes when you are starting a new program or have a new angle on an old program, you can get the newspapers to do a feature story. If this happens, be sure that the story includes how you can be reached. The best story in the world is useless if your address or phone number is not included. On radio, the equivalent of a feature story is a short interview or, better still, a call-in program. Again, it is important that you somehow get in the information on how to contact you. In fact, on radio, this should be done several times, as listeners may not get all the information the first time it is given.

Besides the large mass media, all communities have a number of club, church, and other types of newsletters. Putting your announcement in those targeted to your audience can be both effective and inexpensive. The problem with these is that they usually have a long lead time. Thus, if you want something published the first of January it may have to be in by early November.

Fliers can also be effective if well placed. I have found that good places for fliers are on the cash registers at the local pharmacies, in doctors' waiting rooms, at public libraries, in beauty and barber shops, and in local markets and shops.

One final and excellent source of publicity is word of mouth. To utilize this, let past participants know about future programs. Ask them to post fliers in places that they frequent and also to tell their friends. We have found this to be one of the very best sources of publicity.

Once you have gone through all the trouble of putting your publicity in many places, it is nice to know what is effective. The easiest way of doing this is having a place on your application for people to write in where they found out about your program. In this way you can track your publicity and keep using those sources which are effective, while eliminating those that are not.

Reaching the Hard to Reach

One of the biggest problems for many patient educators is reaching patients who are hard to reach. Many times, we consider those people who are not like ourselves or like our regular clients as being hard to reach. Since in English-speaking countries most health care professionals speak English as their primary language, the hard to reach are often defined as those whose primary language is not English. Other groups often defined as hard to reach are the poor and elderly.

In trying to identify ways to reach these groups, a good place to start is by looking at who is reaching them. Where and to whom do they go for information and service? By this we mean, where do they buy their food and clothing and where are their social and sports activities? Why are these services successful when yours are not? At the same time, examine what happens when the 'hard to reach' enter your health care system. Are there people who speak their language and understand their customs? Are your services physically located in a convenient place? Are people treated in a courteous manner? The ultimate question to ask yourself is 'If you were them, would you use your services ?'

In planning your program you also want to ask yourself if you really want to reach them. This sounds harsh, but it is important to consider *before* beginning your outreach efforts. Really wanting to reach them means that you are willing and able to commit the resources, i.e., staff, time and money to develop and maintain services in those communities. If you do not make efforts to provide ongoing funding or you pull out of a community too fast, without helping that community develop resources and maintain the program, bad feelings, tension and distrust are likely to result. This makes it difficult for anyone in the future to work in that community. Therefore, establishing and maintaining good community relations are also important.

The primary rule in trying to reach the 'hard to reach' is to go to them. Don't expect them to come to you. Take some time out to visit the community you want to reach. Walk or drive around and get to know the physical layout. Where do people congregate? Is there a favorite meeting place? For whom and when? You may want to do this more than once, on a weekday or weekend, or even during different times of the day. Talk to the visible people in the community, such as the local shop owners, religious leaders, postal workers, leaders of sports teams, leaders of other recreational or social clubs, etc. Many times these people can be very informative and helpful. They may be willing to provide you with a location for your program or help you identify and recruit other community members to help plan and organize your programs and services. For example, if you want to do a diabetes program for a Mexican-American community, consult first with the community. If it is the Greek population you are trying to reach, try holding the program in a Greek Orthodox Church or at a Greek social club. If you do not have a Greek-speaking health professional in your team, train a bilingual person from the community to give the course. As a health professional, you can act as the backup consultant.

Also, every community has people whom others turn to for advice. These people are called opinion leaders. Many times, these leaders are not highly visible; however, they are the respected community leaders. Identifying these opinion leaders involves some work. Start by asking ten or so people from the population you are trying to reach whom in the community (other than health professionals) they talk to when they have health problems. Then go to all the people identified and ask them the same question. Again, go to everyone they identified and ask the same question. By now you should have a list of many names. Look for the people whose names keep reappearing. These are probably the health opinion leaders for that community. If you can get these people interested in your program, you will probably find your hard to reach population much easier to reach. In fact, you can train these same opinion leaders to deliver your message. We did this in bringing cancer prevention programs to a Mexican-American community. After identifying fifteen opinion leaders, we trained these leaders in cancer prevention techniques, such as breast self-examination and the importance of Pap smears. The opinion leaders then had meetings in the homes, churches, and social clubs of friends and neighbors. All told, more than 4000 Spanish-speaking women were reached in less than six months.

Opinion leaders can also be useful in identifying a community's health needs and in promoting a program. Utilizing members from the community in any and every way possible is important for program success. Their involvement will ensure that the programs or services are appropriate and relevant to that community's health needs.

Opinion leaders can also be great teachers. If they trust you, they can serve as cultural interpreters. If you let them become your guide, you can avoid many of the problems associated with working with different and diverse groups or cultures. They can help you better understand their community's customs, in particular, their use of language and their concept of time. These, believe it or not, are important when working with people from different cultures or ages.

First of all, none of us likes to learn from someone we do not trust. When cultures, ages, or races differ it is harder to build trust. Often small tests are made to judge someone's trustworthiness. For example, if we ask someone to call us back tomorrow and they do not do it until a week later, they have probably failed our test. People do not usually set up these tests intentionally. Rather, they are a built-in part of doing business. When working in a new community, it is very important that you do not fail these tests. Meet with people on their ground, not yours. This shows your willingness to go to them. If you make commitments be sure to keep them. Never make a commitment you cannot keep. If offered food, eat it. Food is important in all cultures and accepting food shows some acceptance of the culture. If you are invited to a special event, go even if it is not during working hours. Again, this shows that you have some interest in and commitment to the community.

Also, pay attention to the language and words you use. Sometimes programs may have to be renamed because when translated, the meaning changes. For example, the model of car called Nova is difficult to sell to Spanish-speaking people because in Spanish the two words 'No va' mean 'It doesn't go'. Therefore, it is worth the effort to learn the meaning of words before naming your program or when translating your message. You might consider having the community you want to reach name the program; this way they may feel that this is truly their program.

Be aware of how the group you are trying to reach uses time. In some groups it is very important to start exactly on time. In fact, for many groups of older people, everyone shows up fifteen minutes early, so it is best not to wait until the last minute to set up your room. On the other hand, for some cultures, showing up on time would be an insult. Everyone knows that a dinner invitation for 7:00 pm can really mean 7:45 pm! If you show up at 7:00, your hostess will be very embarrassed and probably will not be ready. You can use your cultural interpreter to help find out what 'being on time' means. In planning your program, do not expect the hard to reach to conform to your ideas of time. Rather, plan your program to conform to theirs.

Sometimes the problem is that people do not know your services exist.

You cannot expect the same media messages to get to all populations. If you are trying to reach the elderly, put the information in senior citizens' newsletters and in other publications read by older people. Placing your notice on the same page as the obituaries may sound morbid, but it will get read by the elderly who are looking to find names of friends who have passed away. Find out how news is spread in the community you are trying to reach. It may be that announcements at church or before the community bingo game are effective. If there are special foreign language radio broadcasts or other types of media, do not hesitate to use them. These people are often very eager to help you with publicity.

As was stated at the beginning, the hard to reach are that way because you do not know how to reach them. Using some of these ideas should make this task easier. However, if you find that you are too uncomfortable working in these hard to reach communities, then it is best that you do not. It does not mean you are a bad person. We all have our own prejudices and some are easier to overcome than others. If you are unable to deal with your discomfort in a particular community, you may try to reach out by finding another health professional who has had experience or is more comfortable working with that group.

Utilizing Community Resources

Every community has resources. Finding them is the problem. Sometimes the problem is not really finding them but rather seeing what is before your eyes. For example, every community has hotels, bars and restaurants. However, we seldom think of these as sites for patient education. In fact, many of these establishments spend a great deal of their time nearly empty. Thus, you might be able to use a bar or a restaurant for a morning class. These sites might be especially attractive if you are trying to reach men. Hotel swimming pools are used heavily in the early morning and in the evenings. However, in between times, it might be used for a water exercise class.

In the same vein, doctors all have empty waiting rooms when patients are not being seen; these might be used for evening classes. One elderly group walks inside a shopping mall two mornings a week from 8:00 to 9:00, and then has coffee and a health lecture in the mall coffee shop. Since there are few people in the mall as the shops open at 9:00, the owner is pleased to get the extra business. Another possible site for walking programs is the airport. In large cities, airports have miles of climate-controlled corridors that are good for walking.

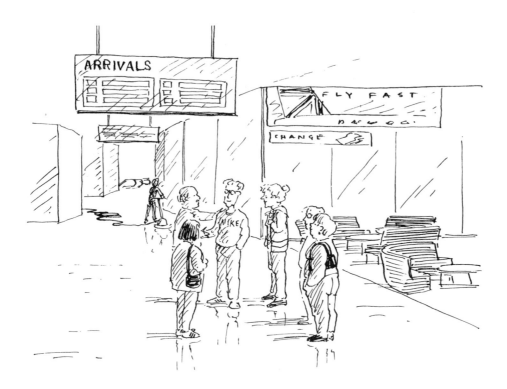

Service clubs are also common in most communities. Lions, Rotary and Elks are all groups which can be called upon for help. One of the missions of these groups is community service. With a little creative thinking, you can help them fulfill their mission. Members of these organizations can be recruited to get people to courses or to give public lectures. Also, most communities have a variety of youth groups, such as Scouts and 4-H. Members of these organizations can be trained as peer counsellors or as babysitters for handicapped children or adults. They are also experts at distributing fliers or announcements. As a special project, they might even design some of your patient education materials. Give them a chance to do their daily good turn.

In large communities, it is often difficult to get access to the media. However, just the opposite is sometimes true in smaller towns. Newspapers and radio stations need material. You may arrange for a weekly newspaper column or to do a stress management program twice weekly over the radio. You will never find out what you can get if you do not ask.

Most merchants are constantly asked for things. Try asking for something different. For example, in a big city ask a major department store to help you advertise an event. In turn, you can go through the store and help them identify those products which they can feature for pregnant women, the elderly, the handicapped, etc. Thus, you are helping them to increase their customer base.

In places that are either very hot, cold, or wet, walking and other outdoor exercises are sometimes a problem. Most of these same communities also have enclosed areas, be they malls, office buildings, airports or markets. Such places can be used for walking programs in the hours before opening. In fact, walking tracks can be marked out with colored tape. Once around the mall equals half a mile or two flights of stairs equals a 20-foot elevation gain.

You can find skilled personnel in much the same way you find sites for your program. Many communities have volunteer bureaus. If you have special needs, ask. There are lots of people who would volunteer if they did not have to lick envelopes or be president of something. If there are no volunteer bureaus, make your needs known through church bulletins or the local newspaper. You never know what will happen.

All the above is fine and good, but what if what you really need is money? The place to start is near home. Ask service clubs, churches, and merchants. Most of these organizations have planned giving programs so they are not going to instantly hand over cash. However, if you understand their programs and how to ask for money through their channels, you may well get what you need. Beyond local organizations, look to governmental groups: local, state or national. Again, there are all kinds of rules and regulations. However, if you are willing to play the game and have a good product, you may well get the funding you need. In dealing with bureaucracies, remember to play by the rules: dot all the i's and cross all the t's. Be sure that the government officials who will fund your request understand your program and are sold on it. After all, they will be the ones to present it to the people higher up. Finally, have enough time. You probably cannot find the funds you need in a week. However, any program which is worth doing today is probably also worth doing in six months.

No matter what you are asking for, one of the best ways to get it is by asking the person or organization you are approaching how to get what you want, the principle being that people usually want to be helpful. For example, if you want the local radio station to air a stress management series, ask the manager what you would need to do to get such a series on the air. He will then outline a number of things for you to do. Listen carefully and write these down. Then do just what he says. If you do this, it will be very difficult for him to keep the series off the air. When someone tells you how to do something and you follow through, they have almost committed themselves to do it.

In short, all communities have resources. Your job is to recognize, find and, most importantly, utilize them effectively.

References

'How-To' Guides on Community Health Promotion
Stanford Health Promotion Resource Center
1000 Welch Rd., Palo Alto, CA 94304

The following guides are available for $2.00 each:

'How-To' Modules

• Volunteers	No. HTP 1	$2.00
• Focus Groups	No. HTP 2	$2.00
• Placing Newspaper Ads	No. HTP 3	$2.00
• Writing and Sending Press Releases	No. HTP 4	$2.00
• Gaining Access to Media Resources	No. HTP 5	$2.00
• Working With Media Gatekeepers	No. HTP 6	$2.00
• Print Production: Dealing With Vendors	No. HTP 7	$2.00
• Building a Media Resources Inventory	No. HTP 8	$2.00
• Conducting a Community Resource Inventory	No. HTP 9	$2.00
• Online Data Retrieval	No. HTP 10	$2.00
• Writing Effective Survey Questions	No. HTP 11	$2.00

Also available from the same address: Gonzales VM, Gonzales JT, Freeman V, et al: *Health Promotion in Diverse Cultural Communities*, Stanford, Calif, Stanford Center for Research in Disease Prevention, 1991.

CHAPTER
5

Helping People
Who Are Hard to Help

One of the greatest challenges in patient education is dealing with people who are hard to help. Thankfully, there are a limited number of problems which seem to appear over and over again. Once you recognize each problem and its solution, dealing with these problems becomes much easier. In this chapter, you will meet some of these people and discuss ways of helping them.

I. The Strong Silent Type

One of the greatest fears of patient educators is that they will not be able to get people to ask questions or to discuss topics. There is also a strongly held belief that says: 'People here are different. They don't talk.' 'Here' can mean any region, country or culture.

People are not really all that different. Rather, it is the patient educators who are insecure about their own knowledge and abilities and never really invite participation. Usually they give a talk and then ask if there are any questions. Given ten seconds and no response, they decide that there are no questions and continue or end the session.

In trying to get participation there are several techniques which are very helpful. You might present a problem or question, such as our old friend, 'What would you do if...?' Have all the participants write down their answers. Then go around the room having each participant tell what he or she wrote. This technique ensures that everyone participates in a non-threatening way. But, in using this technique, first be sure that the question is one which is non-threatening and with which the participants have 'experience'. For example, 'What is the greatest problem in controlling your diet?' When using this technique, the leader should start by modeling an appropriate response using a personal experience. Finally, start with a participant who you know will be able to respond. Once the group is clear on the expectation, then generally everyone will follow.

A second way of getting group participation is to brainstorm. The details for this technique are discussed on page 41.

When asking the group questions, be sure that the question is open-ended. A good rule to follow is never ask a question which can be answered by yes or no. 'What questions do you have?,' not 'Are there any questions?' Then, after asking for questions, count to 30 slowly. Groups do not like silence and someone will generally say something to fill the void. If the silence makes you uncomfortable, then you can add a second prompt like, 'Surely there are some questions?' Once the ice is broken, then more questions and discussion usually follow.

Make the group safe for questions and discussions. Give reinforcement to everyone who participates either with smiles, nods of your head or positive comments, such as 'That is a good question', or 'I'm so glad you asked that. Many people have the same problem and are afraid to discuss it.' Be careful not to make participants feel stupid or silly. Even if you get an off the wall comment, respond with a noncommittal, neutral statement like 'that's an interesting comment' or 'I see your point of view.'

By using the above techniques you can almost always get good group participation. However, there may still be some non-participating group members. First, be sure that these people are sitting in the group. Often they will place themselves physically outside the group. If someone is a chronic non-participant, address questions directly to him or her. For example, 'Jim/Maria, what do you think about that?' Be sure that you do not put the non-participant on the spot. Always ask something that you know he can answer.

Sometimes you will have a situation where a husband or wife answers for their spouse or a parent answers for a child. In this case, address your questions directly to the child or silent spouse. If someone else answers say, 'No, let Jill speak for herself.' Then be patient and let

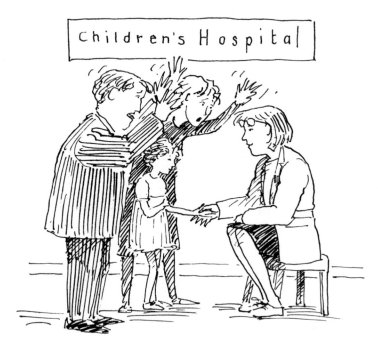

this happen. Be especially sure to reinforce any participation by your strong, silent types. In addition, watch them carefully for any sign that they might like to participate but are holding back. A change in posture, facial expression or slightly raised finger may be all the clue you get. Do not miss these.

In almost every class you will have a sleeper. Do not let this worry you. Just let the person sleep. They are probably tired. It has nothing to do with your presentation. If more than 25% of the class is sleeping, then you might be the problem. However, if the class is made up of medical students or doctors, even a 50% sleep rate is acceptable.

II. The Talkers

Once you get your group to participate, the problem will probably be shutting them up. Too much participation can be just as bad as no participation; this takes skill to control. Here are some situations which might arise.

Participants come to a course with some special problem or question. They often want these answered right away. As a leader, you can easily be thrown from your agenda by trying to meet participants' needs immediately. Do not be afraid to say, 'We are going to discuss medications in the third session. Right now we are discussing exercise.' Or 'That is a little off the topic but I will be pleased to discuss it with you during break. Right now it is important to get on with the class.' To help keep this situation from occurring, you should have an agenda posted at the start of each class, divided into topics and with the time allowed. Then if you are behind you can use the agenda as a reason for charging ahead.

One of the most troublesome of all class participants is the talker. She almost always has something to say which usually includes a long story. Sometimes her stories and insights are very useful and relevant and other times they are useless. In either case the person who usurps time must be controlled. One way to do this is just not to call on the person. However, this is of limited usefulness as this person will often butt in, asked or not. Sometimes you have to be very blunt. 'Your opinions are helpful but others need a chance to be heard.' This may seem harsh and unfeeling; however, such a statement is usually handled with good grace. The people who hog time know when they are being 'hoggish'.

Another frequent problem is when a participant rambles on and on. The point of the story, if there is a point, was made in the first fifteen seconds. In this case, the only thing to do is cut the person off. Wait until he takes a breath—it has to happen sometime—and quickly say, 'Thank you very much.' Immediately call on someone else or start a new activity. Radio talk show hosts are excellent at this.

Side talkers are very common. These are people who are always chatting to their neighbors. To begin with, ask them to be quiet. If this does not work, sit between the two friends. This is sometimes successful. If not, then a little sarcasm might be helpful: 'If you two don't stop talking I'll have to ask one of you to stand in the corner.'

On very rare occasions you will find a whole class that is very difficult to control. They all talk at once. In this case seating can come to your rescue. Although we generally like to have small groups sit in a circle, sitting people in rows, in desks or with tables in front of them tends to reestablish control and quiet discussion. If all else fails, rearrange the room. Of course, if the problem is lack of participation in a formal setting, try making the setting less formal.

III. The Antagonistic or Belligerent Participant

Thankfully, these people do not appear too often. They, too, can be helped. The first thing to remember is not to argue. This just leads to more argument. Instead, try: 'I understand your beliefs but our current knowledge in this suggests...' or 'If you find eating fish cures your ulcers, then please continue eating fish. However, for most people we find that...will be more helpful.'

Sometimes a leader and a participant will get into it with each other. Somehow, whatever the leader says adds more antagonism. When this happens it is usually a play for power from someone who is used to being the center of attention. One way to help this situation is to place the powermonger out of direct eye contact. In a circle, the best way of doing this is to place the person next to the leader. Somehow, being out of eye contact tends to defuse the situation.

If all else fails, you might have to ask the belligerent person to leave the class. This can be done by saying, 'I don't think this class will meet your needs. If you will see me after class or call me tomorrow, we can see if we can find something more suitable.' At this point the belligerent person may leave. More likely, she will simmer down and participate more appropriately. In either case, things will be easier for you and for the participants.

IV. Yes, Buts...

These are the people who always have an excuse for not doing what you ask. They are usually easy to identify by their distinctive call 'Yes, But...' After hearing two to three Yes, Buts, give up. There is no way you can help them by being helpful. Rather confront them, 'I know that you have many problems. However, the decision to do something or not is yours. I don't have high blood pressure so it is not my problem. If you want to do something, fine; I'll try to be helpful. If not, that is OK too. It's your choice.' Such a statement makes it very clear where the problem lies and that it is up to the individual to take responsibility. Do not spend all your time with these people. You probably will not be able to help them. In trying to help them, you deny help to others who are more ready to act. One of the best ways of turning a Yes, But around is to ignore him or her. Often, when you get attention for action rather than non-action, you see a change in behavior.

The 'Know-It-All' is just a variation of the Yes, But. This person knows all the answers and has tried everything. There is nothing you can teach him. Acknowledge that the person is very knowledgeable and that you might not be able to teach him anything. Then give him the choice of continuing or leaving. Most of the time, once the game is called, the person will become an active and helpful participant. Sometimes he will leave and this is OK too.

V. Attention Seekers

We have already talked about several types of attention seekers – the Belligerent, the Know-It-All and the Yes, Buts. There are two more types which, unfortunately, have a high prevalence in patient education classes.

The Whiners are those people with a million problems. Sometimes they are also Yes, Buts. Somehow, they manage to get the whole class involved in the catastrophe they call life. Everyone feels sorry for them. Often their stories are truly traumatic—they were molested as children, have alcoholic husbands, or are about to get evicted from the family home. Besides, no one loves them. First, you must remember that the story may or may not be true. Second, there are probably three or four other people in the class with equally wrenching lives who somehow are coping and productive. If you and the class get bogged down with them, no one wins and everyone loses. Instead, suggest that you will talk with them at break or after class and try to make some appropriate referrals. Do not spend class time in trying to solve their problems!

The second attention seeker plays a game called, 'My disease is worse than your disease.' They seek status by having the worst disease. It is important to cut this game short at the beginning. Statements such as the following may help. 'In this class everyone has problems with... Some of these may seem worse than others, but you can never judge another by your own standard. The paraplegic in a loving family may get along very well, while the loss of a finger can be devastating to a concert violinist. In this class we will try to help everyone with his or her problems and not make judgments about the severity of the problems.'

Another way of cutting short this disease status game is not to let participants give their disease history or to describe themselves in terms of the disease. This is especially important in introductions. Ask people to tell about their families, hobbies or what they want to get out of the course, but *do not ask* them to tell about their disease.

VI. Special Problem People

There are two final types of problems which are not very common but which need to be recognized and dealt with quickly: the 'ists' and the 'inappropriates'.

The 'ists' are the people who are racists, sexists or ageists. They are the men who call women girls, the young people who make rude remarks about older people, and those who use terms like Niggers and Japs. Any time you encounter an 'ist' you should make it clear that such language and thinking does not have a place in this setting. This is true even if you do not have Orientals or older people in your class.

In some ways, the 'inappropriates' are the easiest to handle. These are the people who clearly have a mental health problem that is usually obvious in the first few minutes of the class. If the speech and behavior of the person is not disruptive, then let him or her stay. However, if he or she is in any way disruptive, then help them find a more appropriate setting to work on their problems. It is not fair to the rest of the class to keep such a person around. Again, everyone including the inappropriate person loses.

So far you have visited the most common problem people. Sometimes you may encounter other problems or a group of people with multiple problems. In this case, seek some help. A psychologist or social worker who has experience with group work can be an excellent resource. When you are in trouble, do not be afraid to ask for help.

How Do I Get
People to Do
What Is Good for Them?

Virginia Gonzalez
and
Kate Lorig

SPECIAL PROBLEM OF COMPLIANCE

Various authors and studies have estimated that people comply with new health behaviors 30 to 70 % of the time. On face value, this paints a sorry picture and suggests that compliance is a major problem. However, it is necessary to examine this issue a bit more closely.

For some health related regimens, compliance is a very important issue. We know that it is necessary for many people to take insulin daily in order to control diabetes. However, we do not have any similar data to suggest the type, amount or duration of exercise necessary either to prevent or overcome the musculoskeletal problems caused by arthritis. In her discussion of exercise 'sacred cows', Carolee Moncur points out that we have little scientific information about the number of repetitions or the frequency of either range of motion or isometric exercises needed for therapeutic effects (Moncur, 1988). Thus, much of arthritis physical therapy is built on tradition, common sense, and experience. However, it is not backed by strong scientific evidence. When such evidence is lacking, it is difficult to justify the importance of exact compliance with an exercise program.

Another issue involves the interactions between the disease and the desired health behaviors. For many diseases, the symptoms wax and wane on almost a daily basis. Therefore, the continuation of a set of behaviors in the face of changing symptoms does not seem to make a great deal of sense. Rather than strict compliance, a person must understand the rationale for his or her program and also know how to make daily adjustments in the face of these changing symptoms. If this is not done, behavior change becomes a frustrating experience in which the patient either exacerbates the symptoms or gets no therapeutic effect because the intervention is not tailored to the symptoms. Balancing behavior change with symptoms takes knowledge of, and practice with, decision making skills. Unfortunately, decision making skills are seldom taught in traditional health professional/patient programs.

Based on the above discussion, it would seem that specific compliance may not always be a desired or even necessary behavior. A more appropriate goal might be the adherence to a long term program which changes constantly in response to symptoms. However, even with this broader definition, it is doubtful that most people adopt new programs appropriately. The rest of this chapter will discuss reasons for inappropriate compliance patterns, ways of identifying problems with individual patients, and suggestions for solving these problems. The terms compliance and adherence will be used interchangeably.

Let us now turn to exploring how to help people with compliance. This will be done by use of the decision chart on page 102. Start at the top and work through until you find a description of the problem you are encountering. Each level of the chart has one or more explanations of actions which might be taken. These are indicated in the triangles. Look up the appropriate number and letter to find possible solutions to the problem.

1. Can the patient tell you why he/she is not complying?

This may seem like an obvious question. However, all too often we forget to ask. When we do ask, the patient will usually tell us the problem. The normal response of most professionals when confronted with a patient problem is to offer the patient a solution. This is probably not the best response. Rather, this is an ideal time to teach problem solving skills. To do this, ask the patient to brainstorm possible solutions. For example, if the patient says he does not have enough time to exercise in the morning, ask when else in the day he might have ten minutes to do his exercises. If the patient says he forgets to exercise, ask about activities which are done daily such as reading the morning paper or watching a favorite TV show, then link the exercises to that activity. The moral here is that most patients can tell you the problem and, with a little assistance, come up with a solution. Never underestimate your patient.

2. Is compliance important?

This may seem like a silly question. However, as discussed earlier, we really don't know exactly which exercise program is best for which patient. The result is that we often ask patients to do things which may not be important. For example, are daily range of motion exercises necessary for every stroke patient? The answer is probably no. In fact, range of motion exercise three or four times a week is probably sufficient. Do all joints need to be put through a daily range of motion exercise? Again, the answer is probably no. One needs to exercise only those joints which are not exercised in daily activity and in which there is some limitation. If compliance is not important then forget about it. You and the patient have more important things to worry about.

3. Does your patient believe that compliance will help? (No)

If the answer is no, then the reason for noncompliance is obvious. Why should anyone do anything in which he or she doesn't believe? While the problem may be obvious, the solution is a bit more difficult. People's beliefs are almost always rational, based on past experience, conversations with others or what they have been taught. Often it is the use of language that leads patients to false beliefs. Arthritis health professionals often talk about osteoarthritis as a 'wear-and-tear disease'. It isn't. When heard by patients this idea is easily translated into rational action. 'Why should I exercise if my disease is caused by wear-and-tear? Exercise increases the problem.' One of the ways to help to change beliefs is to change the use of language.

Another means of changing beliefs is to expand on one's current belief system. If someone believes that pain is due to disease, then the way to counter the pain is through medical interventions such as use of medication. However, if one expands his or her explanation of pain to include not only the disease but also pain caused by muscle tension, fear and depression, then other pain management modalities, such as exercise and relaxation, might be tried.

Finding out patients' beliefs is not difficult—ask them. Good questions include, 'What do you think causes your pain?', 'Why is exercise important?', or 'When you think of diabetes, what do you think of?' Before giving any explanation, it is important to find out what the patient already knows and believes. In this way teaching is targeted and time is not wasted. More about beliefs on page 5.

4. Does the patient understand? (No)

Don't believe that a patient understands just because he says he does. This is especially true with medication regimens. It is one thing to repeat what the doctor says and quite another to integrate medication taking into one's daily regimen. The patient is not sure what he is doing; he will often do nothing rather than risk doing something that is wrong.

Any time a patient is given instructions, four steps should be taken to ensure understanding: (1) Tell the patient what you want him to do in plain English. Forget all the terms like 'TID'. (2) If you want the patient to do something, show him what you want him to do and have him return the demonstration until he can do it easily without coaching. (3) Give the patient written instructions, including, if necessary, pictures. (4) Ask the patient to describe what he is going to do. Do not accept a parroting of your original explanation. Rather, ask questions like, 'When are you going to take your medicine and how many pills will you take each time?' In short, TWA—tell, write, ask.

5. Does the patient have the skill to comply? (Yes)

5A. Is compliance punishing? (Yes)

In many cases, complying with health regimens is not only non-rewarding, it is punishing. For example, many drugs have side effects, diets take away pleasures, and exercise may leave one stiff. Each of these cases is a bit different, but the solution is similar. Make compliance less punishing and more rewarding. When compliance means physiological punishment, such as the side effects of chemotherapy or other medications, the use of symptom reinterpretation is useful. See more about this on page 116. Explain that the losing of one's hair means that the medication is working as it is killing rapidly growing cells.

In another case, exercise might be punishing because of the time of day or weather conditions. Few people like to walk a mile on a cold winter day before breakfast. In this case, another time might be found, or a warm place such as a shopping mall, or even an alternative exercise such as riding a stationary bicycle.

5B. Is noncompliance rewarding? (Yes)

Sometimes noncompliance brings rewards such as attention, albeit nagging, from spouses or friends. Also, the short term rewards of noncompliance, such as eating chocolate cake, might outweigh the long term rewards of weight loss. If noncompliance is rewarding, the best thing to do is to remove the reward. Ignoring noncompliance may be difficult but may also be the best way to bring about improvement. This is especially true with couples where sometimes the only communication is nagging. Reestablishing more positive communication patterns may be the answer. Sometimes a compromise is the answer: eat one piece of chocolate instead of a chocolate cake.

5C. Is the behavior too complex? (Yes)

Sometimes we ask patients to do many things all at the same time. They are taking several medications, are on a special diet, and have three sets of exercises to perform daily. In addition, they are asked to have appointments with one or more health professionals on a regular basis. Is it any wonder that they don't comply? Before talking to a patient about compliance, it is important to get the whole picture of what he or she is trying to do. Ask him, 'What are all the things that various people have told you to do?' This may range from flossing teeth to drinking warm milk before going to bed every night. What you want them to do is only a small part of the total picture, and compared to some other activities may be relatively unimportant. In any case, as a health professional, your job is to sort out the jumble and to simplify the regimen. This may mean contacting other health professionals to see which of their instructions are really important. In some cases, the instructions may even be contradictory. For example the rheumatologist says to limit weight bearing exercise because of bad knees, but the cardiologist says to forget the knees and walk as much as possible. The patient loses no matter what he does. Once he understands the whole regimen, then priorities can be set and complexities simplified.

5D. Does the patient forget? (Yes)

This is probably one of the greatest causes for noncompliance. It is not easy to add a new activity to our lives, especially if this activity must be performed more than once a day. There are lots of memory aids, such as setting an alarm clock or wrist watch to remind us when it is time to take medications.

Another and more powerful memory aid is to link the new behavior with an already established activity. For example, range of motion exercises can be done in the morning shower. Medication can be taken when brushing teeth. Most of us are creatures of habit. The easiest way to establish a new habit is to link it with an existing habit.

Does the patient have the skill to comply? (No)

5E. Does the patient have the mental capacity to learn the skill? (No)

If the answer is no, you might try some of the tricks under memory aids. However, it is more likely that you will need to find someone to assist the patient. This might be a spouse or other family member, a neighbor or possibly a home health aide or visiting PT. Many older people who live alone are part of an informal helping network of friends and neighbors.

Such networks are especially helpful for the cognitively impaired. Is there someone who can call twice a day to remind the patient to do something? Maybe there is a neighbor who will take a daily walk with the patient. In any case, the answer is usually to find some assistance.

5F. Does the patient have the physical capacity to do the skill? (No)

If the answer is no, then there are several routes to take. First, the activity might be simplified or changed to be within the physical capacity of the patient, so look at ways to make activities less complex. On the other hand, the patient may simply need assistance.

5G. Teach skill, arrange practice and feedback.

If the patient does not have the skill but has the cognitive and physical capacity to learn the skill, then the tricks to compliance are teaching, practice, and feedback. First, the patient must be taught the skill. This can sometimes be done verbally or in writing. However, if there is any unusual physical skill involved, then teaching must include demonstration and practice. You cannot learn to ride a bicycle from reading a book. It is not realistic to expect a patient to learn to inject insulin from written materials. Rather, the patient needs an opportunity for supervised practice and feedback. It is especially important that during the demonstration the patient himself does the whole activity without assistance. This may be very frustrating for the health professional. However, the important thing is that the patient leaves the teaching session confident that he can 'do it himself'. Remember that even the most complex behavior can be broken down into simple, achievable parts.

The final part of teaching a skill is arranging for feedback. This can be provided as part of the demonstration/return demonstration. Compliance is even more likely if the patient has a way of getting his questions answered and receiving feedback when he is at home. This can often be provided by telephone.

6. Does the patient believe that she can do it? (No)

This is probably the key to many compliance problems. Just because someone knows how to do something and even has the required skills, this does not mean she believes she can do it. Many people who are overweight believe that this condition is harmful, know all about exercise and low calorie food, and even know how to exercise and eat appropriately. However, all these beliefs and knowledge are not enough because the person does not believe herself capable of carrying out the program and losing weight. This belief in one's ability to carry out specific behaviors has been labeled by Bandura as perceived self-efficacy (Bandura, 1986). See section on self-efficacy on page 109.

7. What if the patient doesn't want to comply?

Just because you want the patient to do something and know that it is good for her, is no reason she has to agree. Patients have a right to make their own decisions for their own reasons. You should be convinced that the decision is informed; that is, the patient understands your rationale for wanting her to do something. Once this criterion is met, if the patient still decides not to comply, you should honor her decision. Health professionals have a limited amount of time. Often time is wasted trying to work with patients who really don't want help. This is frustrating both to the patient and the health professional. More important, it deprives other patients who can be helped of the health professional's time. Sometimes the best thing to do is to just let a patient go. If this occurs, make it very clear what you are doing. The conversation might go something like this: 'Mrs Jones, I understand that you don't want to lose weight. We have discussed the various reasons why this is important. However, I do respect your decision. If in the future I can help you with a weight loss program, please let me know.' This conversation does several things. First, it lets Mrs Jones know that the decision not to lose weight is hers. Second, it leaves the door open should she change her mind. Finally, it shows your respect for her, even though you disagree with her decision.

In short, if someone does not want to comply you cannot make them. Sometimes you just can't win them all.

Figure 1
Improving Compliance

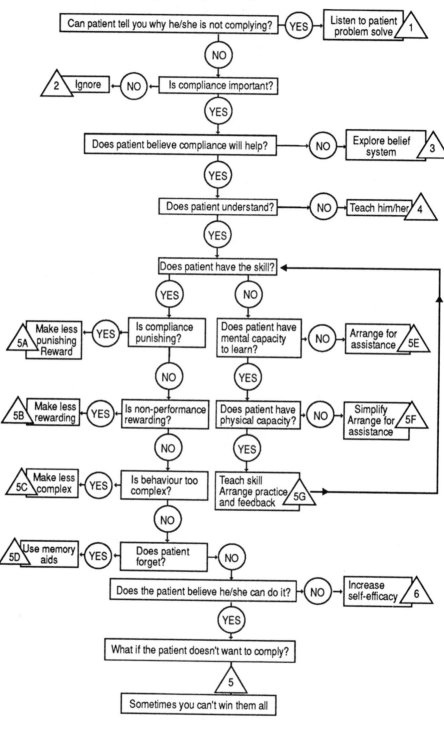

References/Further Reading

1   Bandura, A.,
Social Foundations of Thought and Action: A Social Cognitive Theory, Englewood Cliffs, NJ, Prentice Hall, 1986.

2   Moncur, C.,
'Attacking the Sacred Cows'. *Arthritis Care and Research* 1:2 (116), 1988.

3   Sackett, D.L., Haynes, R.B.,
Compliance With Therapeutic Regimes, Baltimore, The Johns Hopkins University Press, 1976.

What Do We Know
About What Works?

Jean Goeppinger
and
Kate Lorig

PATIENT EDUCATION THEORIES AND MODELS

To make something work, you do not necessarily have to know why it works. Many of us drive cars without understanding how they move. We take medications without knowing how they physiologically affect health. However, a mechanic understands how cars run, and a pharmacist understands how drugs work.

As a patient educator, you can create a program without knowing why it works. However, the strongest programs are based on tested models and theories. In this chapter, we will examine two models and three theories. Most importantly, we will give a rationale or context for patient education. Before going further, let us define terms. A *rationale* is a statement of *reasons*. *Models* are *schemata*, structures for organizing things, while *theories,* considered here, are systems of ideas used to *explain changes* such as improved self-care behaviors or health status.

Rationale: The Compression of Morbidity

For the authors, the best overall reason for patient education is provided by the rationale-compression of morbidity. This provides the foundation upon which all patient education is built. Let us examine this further. In 1981, Dr Fries and Dr Crapo published their book *Vitality and Aging*, in which they argued that the human life span is finite (Fries & Crapo, 1981). That is, no matter what improvements we make, the average human being will probably not live more than 85-95 years. The future will not be peppered with 200-year-old persons. If this is true, then the primary purpose of all health care today is to reduce premature morbidity and mortality rather than to prolong life. Fries and Crapo have termed this 'rectangularizing the curve,' or compressing morbidity. Let us examine some examples to understand this further.

At the present time, someone is born and, barring anything unusual, lives a pretty healthy life until well into the fifth or sixth decade. At this point, we can encounter any of a number of chronic illnesses: hypertension, diabetes, heart disease, osteoporosis and arthritis to list just a few. These illnesses are associated with increased morbidity and compromise an individual's quality of life. The person's health generally declines for the next fifteen to thirty years until death (see Figure 1).

To say that we are going to prevent death from heart disease or diabetes may be unrealistic. However, we may be able to compress

107

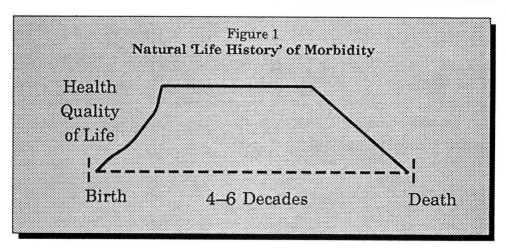

Figure 1
Natural 'Life History' of Morbidity

morbidity. That is, instead of getting a disease at 60, and living with chronic problems for twenty years, we may be able to push disease onset back to 75, thus flattening the curve or compressing the morbidity. Even when someone has an illness, such as heart disease or hypertension, we might be able to stabilize the condition rather than having it progress on a steady downward path. Again, this flattens the curve or compresses morbidity (see Figure 2).

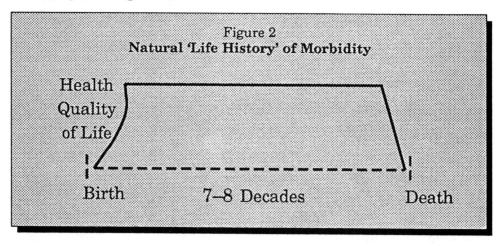

Figure 2
Natural 'Life History' of Morbidity

This can be done with patient education as well as with medical management. Thus, the rationale for health promotion and patient education is to allow people to live the fullest life possible for the longest possible time and to compress the time that they are infirm due to ill health. Now that we have a reason for doing patient education, let's examine some theories and how they might be applied to real world practice.

Three Theories

The purpose of a theory is to provide an explanation of why things happen. If such an explanation is accurate, if we do things similarly a second time, the result should be the same as the first. Theories make the world a much less chaotic place. For example, if we drop a plate, it will fall and probably break. Knowing this, we do not have to keep dropping plates to see what happens. The same is true in patient education. Our theories are far from perfect, but we do know some things. For example, Hougland has taught us that when trying to persuade someone of something, it is often better to give both sides of the argument, instead of just one (Hougland, 1957). In short, the wise use of theory helps us to make things happen in predictable ways.

There are many theories which can be applied to patient education. These come from the fields of communication, organizational development, sociology, psychology and adult education. The best patient education is an appropriate mix and match of theory. This mixing and matching, like being a good cook, comes from experience. However, we cannot mix and match without knowing what possibilities exist. The three theories to be discussed here — self-efficacy, coping and learned helplessness — were chosen because they have particular relevance to patient education. All these have been used successfully to explain the behaviors of patients and have been used in program development.

Self-efficacy Theory

'Perceived self-efficacy is defined as people's judgement of their capabilities to organize and execute courses of action required to attain designated types of performance. It is concerned not with the skills one has but with judgements or beliefs of what one can do with whatever skills one possesses.' (Bandura, 1986)

In examining this definition, several parts need emphasis. First, self-efficacy is behavior specific. That is, there is no such thing as an efficacious person. Rather, someone may have very high efficacy for getting dressed in the morning but very low efficacy for flying an airplane. In this way, self-efficacy differs from two related constructs: learned helplessness and locus of control, which generally refer to relatively enduring personality traits or attitudes rather than to specific behaviors (Wallston & Wallston, 1976; Seligman, 1975).

Second, self-efficacy deals with our perception or belief that we can

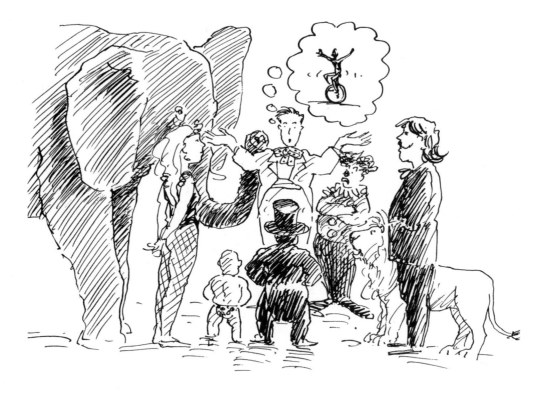

accomplish some future behavior. In this way it is predictive. Our efficacy for future performance is a good predictor of actual future performance. Thus, if I were a circus owner and had to quickly hire a new unicycle rider, I would ask potential employees how certain they were that, given some short instruction, they could ride a unicycle. I would then choose the applicant with the highest efficacy as he or she would be most likely to master quickly the art of unicycle riding.

On the other hand, sometimes there are people who perform quite well but believe that their performance is not up to standard. These people would have low efficacy which, in turn, might prevent them from trying anything more challenging. We often call these people under—achievers. Finally, research has shown us that we can change self-efficacy and that changes in self-efficacy are associated with changes in behavior and cognitive status such as pain and stress. Thus, if we enhance someone's efficacy for not smoking, they are more likely not to smoke. Because of all these characteristics, self-efficacy theory has great applicability to patient education. O'Leary and Bandura (O'Leary 1985; Bandura 1986) have written reviews of research on the use of self-efficacy theory in health. Let us now examine the four specific efficacy enhancing mechanisms which can guide patient education: (1) skills mastery, (2) modeling, (3) reinterpretation of physiological signs and symptoms, and (4) persuasion.

SKILLS MASTERY

Probably the most powerful way of enhancing self-efficacy is through skills mastery. This is generally done by breaking skills into very small, manageable tasks or subgoals and then making sure that each small task is successfully completed. Some of the original work was done with agoraphobics who first walked outside their door, then walked a few steps, then walked to the pavement, etc. Another good example is Alcoholics Anonymous, whose members promise not to drink today. They do not worry about tomorrow. In other words, each commitment or contract is short term, not for life. In devising health education programs, we have found that it is best to have people start with what they are sure they can do now. For example, the person who has had a stroke and who can walk half a block is encouraged to do this four times a week, and then to increase the duration or frequency by not more than 10% each week. Remember that the key to skills mastery is the word *mastery*. It is very important that if people are going to become more efficacious they must be successful in what they are trying to do.

One of the best ways of accomplishing mastery is to have clients contract for specific behaviors. Contracting should be mostly client driven. That is, the client decides on the behavior; it *is not* dictated by the professional. Equally important, there must be an opportunity to give feedback and make mid-course corrections. Every session of a health education course might end with a contracting session and every session begin with feedback on individual performance during the past week. This point is so important that up to 30% of course time may be used profitably in establishing contracts, discussing successes and problems, and providing modifications to behavior change programs.

If education is given on a one to one basis, the feedback mechanism should also be institutionalized. This can be done by noting the contract in the chart and asking about it on the next visit. Better yet is a quick phone call in a week to ten days to see how the contract is going. See the following for an outline on how to do skills mastery contracting.

HOW TO HELP SOMEONE MAKE A CONTRACT

1 Discussing Alternatives

For any problem discuss with the patient the possible behaviors he or she would like to change. If time is short, you might use a prewritten checklist of behaviors. This saves time and ensures you do not forget anything.

2 Deciding What You Want to Accomplish

Ask the person what he or she would like to do this week. This activity should come from them and not you. Note: This point is extremely important.

3 Making a Plan

This is the difficult and most important part of contracting. Part II is worthless without Part III. The plan should contain all of the following elements:

- *Exactly what* is the participant going to do? (i.e. How far will you walk? How will you eat less? What relaxation techniques will you practice?)

- *Once someone has told you* what they would like to do, ask if they have ever done that (i.e. walked two miles) or what has worked in the past (i.e. how have you lost weight in the past?). If someone has never done something before, then they should start on a very simple level. The goal may be to walk two miles, but start with half a mile.

- *When* will you do this? Again, this must be specific (i.e. before lunch, in the shower, when I come home from work). It is best if the new activity is linked to some already established and desired activity, like watching the evening news.

- *How often* will the activity be done? This is a bit tricky. Most participants tend to say every day. In contracting, the most important thing is to succeed. Therefore, it is better to contract to do something four times a week and exceed the contract by actually doing it five times than to contract to do something every day and fail by only doing it six days. To ensure success, we usually encourage people to contract to do something three

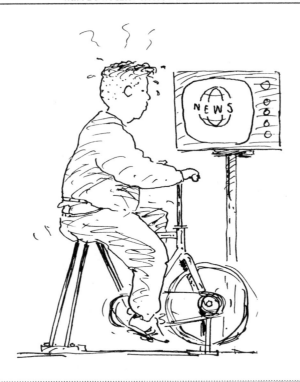

to five days a week. Remember: success and self-efficacy are as important, or maybe even more important, than actually doing the behavior.

4 Checking the Contract

Once the contract is complete, ask the client, 'Given a scale of 0 to 100, with 0 being totally unsure and 100 being totally certain, how certain are you that you will (repeat the participant's contract)?'

If the answer is 70 or above, this is probably a realistic contract and the client should write it down. If the answer is below 70, then the contract should be reassessed. Ask the client: 'What makes you uncertain? What problems do you foresee?' Then discuss the problems. Once the problem solving is complete, have the client restate the contract and repeat as above, checking the contract. Once the clients have settled on a contract, they should write it down. Then each day they should make a check mark if the contracted behavior was achieved. If it was not achieved, they should write a sentence or two about the problems. This record can be used to problem-solve and to monitor progress.

Note: This may seem cumbersome and time consuming. However, it does work and is well worth the effort. Once they learn the format, most clients can contract in less than a minute. Contracting is a learned skill. Thus your clients will soon be saying, 'I will— four times this week before lunch and I am 80% certain I can do this.' One final note: be sure that the clients say '*I will*' not 'I'll *try*'. The latter is not a real commitment.

MODELING

Another excellent way of helping to enhance efficacy and change behavior is to provide opportunities for people trying to change their behavior to see someone else with the same problem. This is the principle used by the American Cancer Society in its Reach for Recovery program, where women who have had mastectomies visit new mastectomy patients. It is also one of the reasons that support groups are so popular and successful. In choosing models you should look for someone who is as much like the patient as possible. Thus matching should be done by age, sex, ethnic origin and socioeconomic status.

Unfortunately, as patient educators, we often use the wrong types of models. For want of a better word, we'll call these 'super achievers'. These are people who have had problems and have overcome them in some spectacular manner. An example would be the marathon runner who lost a leg to cancer, or the older woman with two hip replacements who, after hiking all day, does Scottish dancing. While these people are real inspirations, they are not the best models. Their achievements, to most of us, just do not seem realistic. A better model is someone who has a problem and is coping with it on a day to day basis. This is the type of person to whom your clients can relate.

There are several ways in which to use coping models. You might use lay instructors with the problem. This is the model used by the Arthritis Self-Help Course. Given a structured curriculum, good training, and adequate professional back-up, lay people can make excellent patient education instructors. People with problems can also be brought into health education classes to talk with clients and to share experiences. In one experiment, preoperative cardiac bypass patients were placed in rooms with patients recovering from the same surgery. These patients did better and were discharged earlier than those placed with patients having unrelated conditions.

Another way of using models is to have class members help each other. This is done by allowing the class members, rather than the instructor, to solve problems. Every time a problem is stated, the leader should ask the group if anyone has ever had a similar problem, or has any ideas about how to solve the problem. Class members should also be encouraged to provide feedback. The leader is always the expert of last resort. This teaching strategy has several advantages. First, it teaches class members that they really are experts and have useful knowledge to share. It also teaches them that they do not always have to rely on professionals for expert help. Finally, this approach generates many innovative solutions to problems which would probably never be thought of by professional instructors.

Lastly, all health education media should demonstrate appropriate modeling. This includes videos, tapes, books and pamphlets. If the audience is made up largely of Asians, then the relaxation tape should be recorded by someone from their culture. If you are teaching older people how to get up from the floor after falling, then the pictures you use should be of a slightly overweight older person, not a slim, lithe young woman. Unfortunately, most health education media choose their models

Choose the appropriate role model

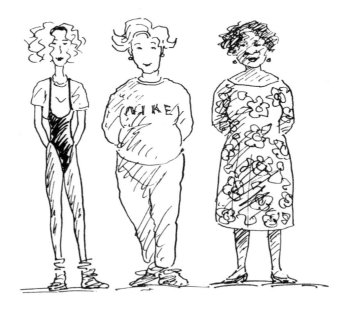

for their photogenic or charismatic qualities rather than for their ability to act as role models.

REINTERPRETATION OF PHYSIOLOGICAL SIGNS AND SYMPTOMS

For the most part, people who are not mentally or cognitively impaired act in a rational manner. At least, their actions are rational within their own belief system. However, as health professionals, we see many actions which do not seem rational. Our job is to determine why people believe as they do and then, when possible, change these beliefs. This is especially true when it comes to disease symptoms. For example, one of the symptoms common to many chronic conditions is fatigue. Patients are usually told to rest or to balance work with rest. It is only recently that we have come to realize that many people with chronic illness are also depressed. Fatigue is a symptom of depression. However, in the case of depression, resting will only exacerbate the fatigue. Therefore, it should be explained to patients that fatigue can come from the disease, in which case resting is a good idea. However, it may also come from depression, in which case exercise may help. Given this explanation, suggest that when people are fatigued, they try exercising. About half the people will find this beneficial and the rest will become more fatigued, in which case they should rest rather than exercise.

Sometimes health professionals give mixed messages. For example, for years we have told people with heart conditions to slow down and take it easy. Is it, then, a wonder that they are confused when we tell them to exercise?

Determining someone's beliefs about a disease is not difficult. All you need to do is ask. Questions which are helpful in soliciting beliefs are: (1) If you stop smoking, start exercising, etc., what are you afraid might happen?, (2) When you think of dieting, cancer, etc., what do you think of? and (3) Why don't you ___?

Once you have identified the belief, you can set out to reinterpret it. Here it is very important to listen to your language. What you say may not be what you mean. In arthritis we talk about 'joint protection' which means using joints in an appropriate, non-stressful way. However, some patients interpret this as not using their joints or protecting their marijuana! Keeping language simple serves everyone's best interests.

PERSUASION

This is the fourth way of enhancing efficacy and probably the way most familiar to health educators. Persuasion has a long history as an educational technique, and can take many forms, from fear arousal to social support. In general, persuasion has been found more popular than effective. One aspect of persuasion which has been found useful is to use health care providers and patient educators to urge clients towards doing slightly more than they are now doing. Goals should be short-term and realistic. Most importantly, they should not be much beyond what the clients believe they can *now* accomplish. Thus, instead of saying, 'You could lose twenty pounds if you tried', it would be better to say 'You could lose 5-6 pounds this month'. It has also been found that physicians' opinions are highly valued. The most important thing a doctor can tell a smoker is, 'I want you to stop smoking', not 'I want you to try to stop smoking'.

In summary, self-efficacy is a person's belief that he or she can perform some future behavior or use some cognitive strategy such as stress reduction. It can be enhanced by skills mastery, modeling, reinterpretation of physiological signs and symptoms, and persuasion.

Coping Theory

It is a generally accepted belief that one of the major functions of patient education is to help patients cope with their need to change health habits or manage illness. However, few patient educators ever look carefully at coping theory literature. The following discussion focuses on the work of Lazarus and Folkman. Although their work is only one of many coping theories (Lazarus & Folkman, 1984) it was chosen because it fits well with self-efficacy theory and has practical applications in the real world.

According to Lazarus and Folkman, coping is defined as 'the person's constantly changing cognitive and behavioral efforts to manage specific external and/or internal demands that are appraised as taxing or exceeding the person's resources.' In other words, coping is all those things people do or think in response to things they perceive as problems.

In examining this theory there are several key points.

❏ First, coping efforts are not constant over time but, rather, are ever changing in response to new situations. Obviously, people cope differently given different situations. For example, a person may have little problem in losing weight, but may be unable to stop smoking. Also, the way someone copes today may be very different from the way someone copes tomorrow, even in similar situations.

117

❑ Secondly, coping efforts are both behavioral and cognitive. That is, people do things and think in different ways in order to meet specific situations. For example, someone goes to a doctor for chest pain but ignores hip pain.

❑ Thirdly, to stimulate coping efforts, the situation must seem taxing or stressful to the individual. The reality of the situation as seen by others has little to do with how a specific person sees the same situation. This is why different people react to the same situation in very different ways. For example, one person may view minor surgery as a relatively unimportant inconvenience, while for another person the same surgery can become a major frightening event. The first person may not need to use any unusual coping strategies, while the second may need to employ many strategies in order to cope successfully.

When examining stress and coping theory, two factors must be considered: the personal factors and the situational factors. The personal factors are all those things that the individual brings to the situation, most importantly his or her personal life experience and history. The situational factors are just that, situational. A lion at the zoo probably does not arouse any stress. Seeing one on a safari in Africa may arouse some excitement but probably little fear. But encountering a hungry mountain lion while negotiating a narrow mountain trail may arouse a great deal of anxiety. In all three cases, the stimulus, a lion, is the same. However, the situations, in this case the physical environments, are very different. The same is true for patients. A fever in a three month old is quite different from the same fever in a six year old. Thus, stress is caused by how the individual sees or appraises both personal and situational factors.

In effect, how a person sees a situation or appraises it is the key to how that person reacts to it. This is similar to our discussion of self-efficacy and how beliefs determine how we react to a specific physiological sign or symptom. See page 109. Appraisal is our way of evaluating a situation and determining whether or not a threat exists.

There are two types of appraisal, primary and secondary. Primary appraisal is a judgment about whether an event creates a sense of harm or loss. The Health Belief Model would call this perceived threat (see page 129). Thus, for someone very concerned with cancer, a breast lump may create a sense of potential harm or loss, while for someone ignorant of the warning signs of cancer, a painless breast lump would be given no significance. Secondary appraisal is the judgment as to whether or not the situation is changeable or controllable. For someone who has seen his/her grandparents live full lives as diabetics, diabetes may seem controllable. For another person who has had a friend die from diabetes, the diagnosis of this disease may be a catastrophic event. The difference is that the first person's secondary appraisal is of a controllable event while the second person sees an uncontrollable event. Secondary appraisal is very much like the expectation step in the Health Belief Model where the individual determines the potential for personal control (Becker, 1974). Self-efficacy can also be considered another way of expressing secondary appraisal.

In planning patient education programs, appraisal can be used to recruit patients and guide program content. For example, if people are concerned about the transmission of AIDS, then an AIDS education program should be advertised as 'How to Avoid AIDS,' not 'New AIDS Treatment'. However, if you are giving a program for AIDS patients, then the second topic may be more appropriate.

So far we have examined how individuals' appraisal of situations influences their responses. Let us now look at the common coping responses used in illness situations. Lazarus and Folkman have identified eight distinct ways of coping. These include confronting, distancing, self-control, seeking social support, accepting responsibility, escape-avoidance, problem-solving and positive reappraisal. This list of responses is not all inclusive and may change depending on which researcher created the list. It is presented here simply to give the patient education practitioner some ideas about the types of coping strategies that might be included when planning health education programs. Each strategy can be either positive or negative, depending on the situation and how it is applied.

❑ *Confronting* is probably not a useful way of dealing directly with an illness, as there is no way an illness can respond. On the other hand, if the problem is another person's actions in face of the illness, then confronting could be a very useful strategy. For example, if a spouse is non-supportive, confronting may be a useful coping mechanism. In this instance, an appropriate strategy would be teaching patients to report their own feelings rather than blaming their spouses about lack of support. When communicating, confrontation can also be used in helping people to take actions on destructive behaviors, such as drinking. Thus,

'Tough Love' is a form of confrontational coping (York, York and Wachtel, 1982).

❑ *Distancing* is the strategy by which people separate themselves from the problem. They somehow convince themselves that their condition is different from anyone else's and, therefore, they cannot benefit from the experience of others. People who distance are those who come to a class or support group and complain because the people in the group are different from them. In some cases, this complaint is realistic. However, in others, it is just a way of saying, 'I am coping with my problem by distancing myself from it'.

❑ *Self-control* is a coping strategy highly encouraged by most health educators. It is taking an active interest in coping with the problem by taking control and practicing such activities as self-care and active decision-making. The one caution with self-control is that if it is encouraged too much it may result in victim blaming. For example, someone who has suffered hemiplegia after a stroke should be encouraged to exercise. However, the stroke should never be blamed on that person's prior lack of exercise. Also, given highly unpredictable or uncontrollable situations, the unfettered use of self-control could lead to learned helplessness. More about this on page 122. One thing clients need to learn is the difference between what they can and cannot control. Trying to control the uncontrollable can be very counterproductive.

❑ *Seeking social support* is a well known coping mechanism. Needless to say, social support is generally considered a useful and productive coping mechanism. When building social support, the perception of having support is probably more important than the objective or actual support received. In other words, someone may have a loving family with lots of support but perceive that they have little support. Another person may have only a little support from a friend but perceive that he has good support. In this case, the second person may cope better than the first. Patient education programs should not only try to build the amount of support but also the patient's perception of their support.

❑ *Accepting responsibility* is a coping mechanism which applies more to business than to illness. Although some illnesses may be due to past actions, trying to get someone to accept responsibility is probably counterproductive and only adds to victim blaming. On the other hand, taking personal responsibility is extremely important when trying to encourage the treatment or preventive practices such as medication taking, smoking cessation or weight loss. Thus, this is a coping strategy which is most useful when used selectively.

❏ *Escape-avoidance,* like other strategies, can either be good or bad. Sometimes, the best thing to do with a problem is not to deal with it. However, in the case of most illnesses this is not possible. Avoidance may be a good short term solution but usually does not work in the long run.

❏ *Problem solving* is one of the most useful illness coping strategies. Unfortunately, most patient education programs teach solutions, not the problem solving process. It is like feeding the starving man a fish instead of teaching him how to fish. The skill of problem solving, therefore, is a coping strategy which should be more utilized.

❏ *Positive reappraisal* is a strategy used successfully by many people with illness. Instead of dwelling on what they cannot do, they work at being successful at what they can do. By looking at an illness as a challenge or opportunity, many people have been able to accomplish things which they would have never done if not faced with the illness. Again this is a strategy which deserves emphasis in health education programs.

Rosenstiel and Keefe have identified the coping strategies used by patients with low back pain as reinterpreting, activity, distraction, self-talk, ignoring and prayer (Rosentiel & Keefe, 1983). Two of these strategies, reinterpreting and ignoring, are old friends. Lazarus and Folkman called them positive appraisal and escape-avoidance. Let us now examine the others.

❏ *Activity* is fairly self-explanatory. Activity is an excellent coping strategy, especially when dealing with pain, depression, or trying to change habits like eating or smoking. This strategy can cover many things, including physical activity such as walking or swimming, or more passive activities like knitting, reading or painting. Generally, doing something is better than doing nothing.

❏ *Distraction* is a coping strategy for pain, depression and changing habits. It works on the principle that the human mind cannot think of two things at the same time. Therefore, if the mind is occupied, pain, depression and other cognitive problems are lessened. Distraction can take many forms including going to see a funny movie or counting backwards from 100 by threes to help insomnia. The principle is that, whatever the activity, the mind must be kept fully occupied. In recent years humor has been used as such a coping mechanism. This is another of the many forms of distraction.

❑ *Self-talk* is a variation on positive thinking. All of us talk to ourselves all the time. For example, 'I don't really want to get up, it is too cold.' Self-talk can be either a negative or a positive coping strategy because it often becomes a self-fulfilling prophecy. In helping clients use self-talk constructively, have them write down the conversations they have with themselves and then change all the negative talk to positive talk. For example, 'I don't really want to get up, but if I do I can read the paper and have a cup of coffee.'

❑ *Prayer* is one coping strategy that is often ignored by health educators. Somehow we feel that this is best left to the individual or to the clergy. However, for certain segments of the population, it is a very powerful and useful mechanism which should be used more often. One innovative use of prayer and religion was made in an arthritis program serving a rural southern population. Many of the justifications for self-help activities were backed with Biblical quotes. Also, if people had a problem with the relaxation exercises, they were instructed to substitute silent prayer.

In conclusion, stress and coping theory provides us with many ideas for use in patient education. Patient educators should take the time and effort to formalize the teaching of coping strategies in their programs. Not all strategies will work for all patients. However, by offering a variety, the chances are greater that individuals will find something of value.

Learned Helplessness Theory

Learned helplessness is a third 'theory' drawn from social psychology which is relevant to healthful behavior change. The theory evolved from the animal research of Seligman and Maier (Seligman & Maier, 1967). They observed that dogs which had learned that electric shock was inescapable, irrespective of their responses, became unresponsive or helpless. In social psychological terms, the dogs learned that shock was 'non-contingent', that it occurred independently of their actions. No matter what they did, they were shocked! 'Non-contingency', the recognition that an event like shock occurs independently of your actions, is considered the basic cause of learned helplessness.

This initial research led to much discussion about the relevance of learned helplessness to human behavior, controversy about the causes of helplessness, and eventually the development and elaboration of the Learned Helplessness Model by Seligman (Seligman, 1975). Seligman's work attempts to understand or explain how non-contingency develops in humans. Three causes or 'causal attributions' have been identified: (1) internal versus external, (2) global versus specific, and (3) stable versus unstable. These three attributions are related but we will look first at each separately.

❑ The first cause distinguishes between helplessness caused by oneself and that caused by other factors. It describes a continuum of attributional style referred to as internality versus externality. The frame of reference used to determine an individual's relative placement on this continuum is the familiar self-other dichotomy. Simply stated, an individual may believe that the reason his actions did not result in the desired outcome could be attributed solely to internal, personal factors such as not exercising enough or eating the right foods. An individual at the opposite end of the continuum may attribute non-contingency to external, universal factors such as the weather or bad luck.

For example, smokers who attribute failure to stop smoking to lack of will power are operating in a personal helplessness mode. They may believe that lack of will power is a fatal personality flaw that will result in inevitable failure. Thus they give up trying. Other smokers may ascribe similar problems to social pressure or genes. These persons are considered to be operating in a universal helplessness mode, emphasizing external causes which may or may not be remediable.

❑ The second cause of helplessness distinguishes between global and specific causes. Global helplessness suggests that learned helplessness occurs across a wide range of situations, from driving a car to holding a job to losing weight. Specific helplessness implies that the problems occur across a narrow range of situations. For example, a person could drive a car and hold a job but be totally unsuccessful at losing weight. Attributing failure to global factors results in helplessness generalizable to other situations ('I cannot drive a car, hold a job or lose weight'). When attributed to specific factors, however, helplessness deficits occur only in the original situation ('I cannot lose weight').

❑ The third cause distinguishes between learned helplessness occurring occasionally or consistently over time. This cause consists of a continuum of stable to unstable attributions. Stable attributions are generally recurrent factors; unstable attributions are short-lived or intermittent factors. We might not, for example, ever be able to lose weight, a stable attribution; we might, however, only be unable to lose weight during the Christmas holidays. Psychologists also call this a trait-state distinction; traits are stable attributes, states are transitory.

The descriptions of attributional style are interrelated. Internal attributions are apt to be more stable and global than external attributions. These links are, however, not always the same and should never be assumed. Thus, an individual's relative placement on *each* of the three continua in a *particular* situation determines his or her degree of helplessness. It also assists in predicting the occurrence of future helplessness problems.

These causal attributions lead to an expectation of failure or lack of control, which, in turn, results in the problem termed 'learned helplessness', that is, a problem in motivation, cognition, and action. Problem-solving attempts occur infrequently; for example, the typical response is 'What difference does it make?' Depression is a common result of learned helplessness.

Learned helplessness encompasses some of the same concerns as self-efficacy and stress and coping theories. For example, learned helplessness includes behaviors as well as thoughts and feelings. Self-efficacy focuses on behaviors, while stress and coping considers thoughts, feelings, and behaviors. The Learned Helplessness Model does not, however, *directly* suggest either appropriate coping behaviors or theory-derived interventions as do self-efficacy and stress and coping theories. On the other hand, it may better explain human responses to some diseases where there is often a notable lack of relationship between most behaviors and resulting clinical outcomes (Lorig & Laurin, 1985). Multiple sclerosis is well known for its unpredictable, even capricious, course of 'flares' or exacerbations and remissions, particularly in its physical manifestations. Unpredictability and capriciousness are close in meaning to, if not synonymous with, non-contingency. This suggests that the use of self-efficacy and, to a lesser extent, stress and coping theories to guide intervention may not be enough. Intervention needs to emphasize cognitive and emotional as well as behavioral ways of handling uncertainty.

THEORY-BASED PRACTICE GUIDELINES

Interventions which may be effective in lessening learned helplessness included strategies similar to those mentioned earlier and derived from self-efficacy and stress and coping theories: skills mastery, modeling, reinterpreting or cognitive restructuring of the signs and symptoms of disease and problem, and emotionally focused ways of coping. Cognitive restructuring may be one of the most important, so it will be reexamined briefly. It is an approach to increasing clients' beliefs in personal control of their interpersonal and social environments.

The critical factor in determining an individual's response is not the actual situation as much as how the person labels or evaluates the situation. This is also the basis of the Health Belief Model (the perceived susceptibility and severity variables). See page 129. If negative emotions occur because individuals unthinkingly accept certain illogical or irrational ideas, then teaching clients to think more logically and rationally might create positive emotional states that, in turn, change behavior in healthful directions. It is, for example, more rational to believe 'I have difficulty in losing weight' than 'I'll never be thin'. 'Difficulties' can be managed; if one can 'never' be thin, change will be unsuccessful!

HOW TO HELP SOMEONE COGNITIVELY RESTUCTURE THOUGHTS

The specific steps of intervention utilizing cognitive restructuring include:

❑ *Helping clients accept the fact that self-statements mediate emotions*

The self-statement 'I'll never be thin' arouses helplessness, whereas the statement 'I have difficulty in losing weight' represents a challenge.

❑ *Assisting clients to recognize the irrationality of certain beliefs*

The patient educator should ask the client to consider: What evidence supports my belief? What parts of my beliefs are true, and what parts are false? Am I distorting events? That is, what data suggest that I will *never* lose weight? Can I lose weight but still not be 'thin'? Is 'thinness' a realistic goal?

❑ *Helping clients understand that the inability to initiate or sustain desirable behaviors frequently results from irrational self-statements*

Negative emotional responses can be maintained easily and indefinitely by irrational thinking. Clients need, among other things, to stop thinking irrationally in order to facilitate constructive behavior change.

❑ *Helping clients modify their irrational self-statements*

Have the client write down rational self-statements and rehearse them in role-playing situations. Imagine presentations of troublesome situations. A colleague's going away party replete with pastries and junk food, for example, can be described to the client by the intervener and rational self-statements can be practiced.

In summary, learned helplessness occurs most frequently in situations where the client believes he or she has little control. The result of helplessness is often depression. Learned helplessness can be overcome by reconstructing thoughts and self-statements.

Two Models

In planning a patient education program, it is necessary to have a rationale and one or more theories. Then you can use a model to put these all together. A model is a conceptual framework or a frame of reference which gives you the outline with which to continue. We will describe two models: PRECEDE and the Health Belief Model (Green, 1980; Rosenstock, 1990). Both have been widely used in health promotion and patient education programs. Again, like theory there is no one perfect model. Rather, you will have to choose the one which best meets your needs.

The PRECEDE Model

The PRECEDE model suggests looking at three factors when planning a patient education program. These include predisposing, enabling and reinforcing factors. All of these will be discussed in detail.

A PREDISPOSING FACTORS

These factors can largely be divided into two categories – beliefs and benefits. Your job is to discover what these are. People generally act in a rational manner – at least, they have reasons for doing what they do, although you may not agree with them. However, there are always reasons. For example, if someone believes that exercise will cause a second heart attack, it is not surprising that he or she does not want to exercise. In the same vein, if someone thinks that taking a medication will have serious side effects, it is no wonder that they do not take the medication.

In order to change beliefs, you must first find out what they are. This can usually be done by asking one of the following questions: 'What do you believe might happen if you——?' (Fill in the blank with the desired behavior, such as take medication or exercise) or 'Why don't you——?' (fill in a health behavior) or 'What do you think causes——?' (fill in the blank with a symptom such as pain).

Once you know a belief you can set out to change it. This can usually be done through explanation. For example, 'I can understand why you might think that muscle relaxing exercises would not help pain. However, when you have pain the muscles in the area become tense. These tense muscles can cause more pain. You can help this in two ways: (1) by strengthening the muscles with appropriate exercise, and (2) by learning how to relax the muscles with muscle relaxation techniques. Would you like me to show you how to strengthen and relax your muscles?'

Sometimes you cannot change a belief. If this belief is very important to the individual or is widely held in the culture, it may be very hard to change. In such cases you may not have to change the belief, especially if it is not interfering with behavior change. Rather, you can add to an existing belief. For example, 'I know that you believe that God cures everything and that prayer is very important. I agree. In Biblical times, Sophocles said, "Heaven never helps the man who will not act." This was later translated by the American Ben Franklin to "God helps them that help themselves." Don't you think that your prayers might work better if you gave God a little help?'

In both these cases, helping someone change or add to their beliefs would be helpful in accomplishing both behavior change and enhancing self-efficacy.

Another predisposing factor which might get in the way of behavior change is secondary gain that can come from having an illness. We may use illness as a reason for not working, getting the family to do chores or as a way of getting attention and sympathy from friends. If this is the case, we have very little motivation for getting better and lots of reasons for not changing behaviors. No behavior change will take place until the benefits are changed. If family and friends ignore illness behaviors but give encouragement to new healthful behaviors, the reward structure changes. This is sometimes a very delicate matter. You must plan a program which includes family members and then work with the whole family to change the benefits.

As a patient educator, you may actually contribute to the problem. For example, some people in patient education classes always have an excuse for not doing something. We sometimes call this a 'yes, but...'. By their actions they force you and other class members to spend lots of time with them. In this case, it is best to cut the person short and spend your time with people you can help. This is discussed more on page 89.

B   Enabling Factors

These are the factors which help people do something which they really believe they should and want to do, but feel they are not able to do. Things such as the complexity of the regimen, distance, lack of skills, or lack of ability get in the way. There are two major ways to enable people: finding resources and skills mastery. Someone may not take part in education or healthful behaviors because they lack time or fiscal resources. In this case your job is to help them understand how they can make the behavior change given their life circumstances, and schedule your educational activities at times and places that make attendance possible. More about this on page 71.

To achieve skills mastery, try not to solve problems but rather teach problem solving skills. Work with the individual to find what is needed. Brainstorm ideas of where the person might find resources, make suggestions about resources, or even look up resources if necessary. Then plan with the individual how he or she will make contact with the resource and how it will be used.

When working with enabling factors, the major objective is to assist the person in gaining control. This is important to keep in mind, as many times people will try to get you to do something which they could well do themselves. For example, do not get trapped into always providing transportation. See if someone else in the class or a family member can do this. Usually, if people want to do something badly enough, they will find a way. By always supplying easy answers, you are reinforcing enabling dependency rather than encouraging self-sufficiency. Sometimes being too helpful can be harmful. In other words, supply information but not direct help, unless it is absolutely necessary.

C   Reinforcing Factors

Once someone has decided to do something, whether they continue doing it is largely dependent on reinforcing factors. These include the support of family and friends, the opinions of their doctor and other health care providers, and the person's satisfaction or dissatisfaction with the results. Again, there is a great deal that you can do to assist with the reinforcement. This includes arranging for the use of modeling, which was discussed on page 114 , and persuasion, as discussed on page 116.

Another very important way of reinforcing behavior change is through inclusion of family, friends and health care providers in your educational efforts. If the family is supportive and the professional health care providers are interested in the behavior changes and encouraging, this can make all the difference. Enlist their aid. Do not ignore these important players in your program planning efforts.

Thankfully, we have one final important reinforcing factor. When patients become a bit more confident and start taking their medicine, exercising or otherwise changing to more healthful behaviors, they feel better. This, in turn, reinforces them to continue doing what they are doing. Healthful change, with its obvious benefits, is self-sustaining!

In conclusion, when planning and implementing the PRECEDE model, examine the predisposing, enabling and reinforcing factors. Once these have been determined, use components from self-efficacy, coping and learned helplessness theories to intervene. For example, if you find that a post coronary patient believes that exertion will cause a second heart attack, and that the spouse shares these beliefs, then the intervention should emphasize reinterpretation of symptoms (cognitive restructuring) for both the patient and spouse. In addition, the patient should be taught exercise skills and asked to write a contract around these skills. The spouse can learn how to be supportive (reinforcing). Both may learn strategies for coping with problems as they arise. Figure 3 is an example of how the PRECEDE model and one theory, self-efficacy, might be integrated.

Health Belief Model

The Health Belief Model is one of the oldest and most widely used health education models. It was originally formulated during the 1950s to explain why people did or did not participate in free tuberculosis screening and prevention programs. Since that time, it has undergone revision and has been used to plan many programs. The basis of this model is that people act based on perceptions. These can be divided into two major classes: perceived threat and expectations. Let us examine these a bit more closely.

Figure 3

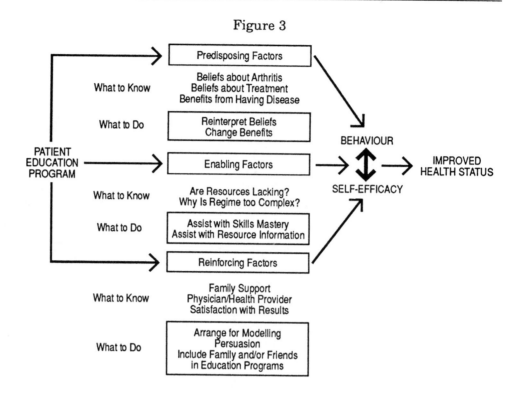

❏ PERCEIVED THREAT

If someone does not see something as threatening, then there is no reason to act. There are two components of perceived threat: perceived susceptibility and perceived severity. Most people perceive AIDS as being a severe disease, not only because of its prognosis, but also because of its severe social and financial consequences. However, there are many different beliefs about susceptibility to AIDS. If one is a sexually active male homosexual, then the belief in susceptibility may be very high. However, if one is a heterosexual living in a middle class suburb, the belief about susceptibility may be low. Thus, while both people believe in the severity, one is more likely to practice safe sex. On the other hand, someone might avoid going to dinner with a friend who has the flu because of belief in susceptibility. However, the same person might get on a bus with someone who might have the flu, thinking that the susceptibility was less.

To change health behaviors, you usually must come to believe in an optional combination of personal susceptibility and severity. This is the reason why many people 'get religion' after they have been diagnosed with cancer or heart disease. At this point, they believe themselves susceptible and, thus, finally give up smoking or lose weight.

❑ EXPECTATIONS

Belief in severity and susceptibility are not enough for new behaviors to occur. People must also have the expectations that: (1) the new behavior will be beneficial in reducing either their susceptibility to or the severity of the condition, (2) the barriers to change do not outweigh the benefits, and (3) one can accomplish the needed behavior change (our old friend, self-efficacy; see page 109).

A kind of cost-benefit analysis takes place on a non-conscious or semi-conscious level. Many people do not like taking medications because of side effects. In the case of headaches, they would sometimes rather have pain than gastrointestinal problems. With hypertension, the problem is more complex because there are usually no symptoms and there may be side effects. Therefore, unless one has a strong belief in severity and susceptibility, the barriers—side effects—can easily outweigh the benefits.

Unfortunately, for many behaviors, the barriers are predictable and immediate and the benefits uncertain and long range. Said another way, the barriers are certain unpleasantness now which needs to be weighed against not so certain future benefits. An example is not eating chocolate

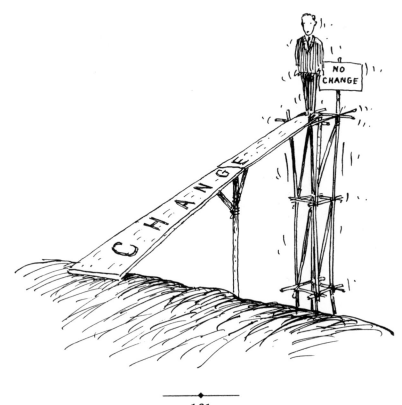

cake now in the hope of avoiding diabetes or a stroke in the future. Looked at this way, it is not hard to see why it is so difficult to get patients to change behaviors. On the other hand, a patient by definition already has a problem. Thus, the cost-benefit ratio is more in favor of behavior change.

Having examined the essence of the Health Belief Model, two more items should be mentioned. To a great extent, our expectations are shaped by background factors (the PRECEDE model would call these factors predisposing; see page 126). Finally, cues to action seem to have an important role in determining if a person actually changes behavior. For example, someone may know that being overweight is unhealthy and that dieting will lower weight. He might also feel he has the skills to lose weight but still nothing happens. During a routine check-up, our mythical person finds he has high systolic blood pressure. This cue moves this person to a weight control program. Cues are elusive; they really cannot be planned. However, by providing patients with examples, and also hints on how to get started easily, we can hope to supply the necessary cue. Of course, some cues are external and hit hard, such as a stroke or the death of a friend from cancer. Unfortunately, we still have a lot to learn about what motivates a person to action. However, providing people with cues seems to be important.

Figure 4

Health Belief Model

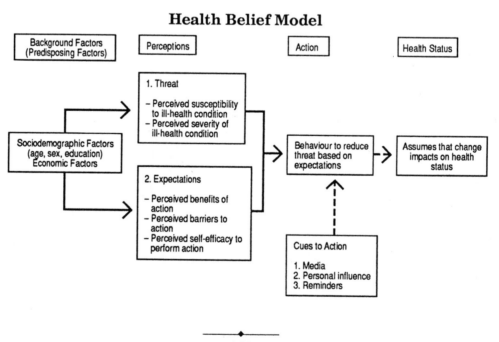

Conclusions

In this chapter we have examined a rationale, three theories and two models which are useful in planning patient education programs. The purpose in providing this material is to give you some tools with which to build a program. Putting together a good patient education program is a little like building a house. You need a grand design. This is provided by the models and theories you choose to incorporate. Will your house be made of bricks, wood, or concrete? Will it have two bedrooms or five? If you do not have a plan in mind, you will probably build a shack. Next, you need the materials — the actual bricks, wood, glass, nails, etc. This is the content of your course, what you are going to teach. Much of this content was determined in your needs assessment. Without quality materials, your building will rapidly become dilapidated. Finally, you need tools. These help you put your materials together in an efficient manner which turns the raw material into the home of your dreams. In patient education, the tools are the processes through which you choose to deliver your content. These processes are discussed in Chapter 3. Just as you would not build a house using just one tool, no matter how useful, you should not build a patient education program using just one process. As a patient educator, you are the contractor. This book has provided you with ways of determining content and designing a plan and a guide to the use of tools. However, like a contractor, the final design and product are up to you. To help you with this design, the following chapter has a check list.

References

1   Bandura, A.,
     'Self-efficacy in Human Agency', *Am Psychol* 37:122-147, 1982.

2   Bandura, A.,
     Social Foundation of Thoughts and Actions: A Social Cognitive Theory, Englewood Cliffs, NJ, Prentice Hall, 1986.

3   Bandura, A.,
     Self-efficacy Mechanism in Physiological Activation and Health Promoting Behavior, Maddon, IO, S. Mathysse and J. Barchas Eds., *Adaptation, Learning and Effect*, New York, New York, 1986.

4   Becker, M., Ed.,
     'The Health Belief Model and Personal Health Behavior', *Health Education Monographs* 2:236, 1974.

---

5   Lazarus, RS., Folkman, S.,
    Stress Appraisal and Coping, New York, Springer, 1984.

6   Fries, JF., Crapo, LM.,
    Vitality and Aging, San Francisco, Calif, W.H. Freeman, 1981.

7   Green, LW., Kreuter, MW.,
    *Health Education Planning: An Educational and Environmental
    Approach*, Palo Alto, Calif, Mayfield, 1991.

8   Hougland, CI., Ed.,
    The Order of Presentation in Persuasion, New Haven, Yale Uni-
    versity Press, 1957.

9   Lorig, K., Laurin, J.,
    'Some Notions About Assumptions Underlying Health Education',
    Health Education Quarterly 12(3):231-243, 1985.

10 O'Leary, A.,
    'Self-Efficacy and Health', *Behav Res Ther* 23:437-451, 1985.

11 Rosenstiel, AR., Keefe, FJ.,
    'The Use of Coping Strategies in Chronic Low Back Pain Patients:
    Relationship To Patient Characteristics and Current Adjustment',
    Pain 17:33-40, 1983.

12 Rosenstock, IM.,
    *The Health Belief Model: Explaining Health Behavior Through
    Expectancies*, Glanz, R., Rimer, B., Lewis F., Eds., *Health Behavior
    and Health Education: Theory, Research, and Practice*, San
    Francisco, Jossey-Bass, 1990.

13 Seligman, M.,
    Helplessness: On Depression, Development, and Death, San Fran-
    cisco, W.H., Freeman, 1975.

14 Seligman, M., Maier, S.,
    'Failure to Escape Traumatic Shock', *Jour of Exper Psych* 74:1-9, 1967.

15 Wallston, B.S., Wallston, K.A., Kaplan, G.D., Maides, S.A.,
    'Development and Validation of the Health Locus of Control (HLC)
    Scale', *Journ Consult Clin Psychol* 44:580-585, 1976.

16 York, P., York, D., Wachtel, T.,
    Tough Love, Bantam Books, New York, Doubleday & Co., 1982.

CHAPTER

8

So Now
What Do We Do?

PUTTING IT ALL TOGETHER

So far this book has dealt with many bits and pieces. However, it may be difficult to put these to use in formulating a patient education intervention. This is rather like turning the raw ingredients of eggs, sugar, flour and chocolate into a chocolate cake. Having the ingredients is not enough. You need a recipe or guide of the amount and order in which you should mix and blend the ingredients. The following is such a guide. It is a checklist of items to be considered in forming a patient education intervention. To use it look at each item and answer, '*Yes*, I'm doing this', or 'This is *not applicable* to me at this time', or '*No,* I'm not doing this and need to know more'.

If your answer is 'not applicable' take a minute to convince yourself that this is really true. While it is true that not every program must go through every step, cutting steps is often a way of fooling ourselves. Unfortunately, there is no easy short cut to patient education. Throwing ingredients together in a haphazard way often results in a rather strange cake.

Finally, if your answer is 'no', there are chapter numbers by each step to help you learn more and move on to the next step.

Putting It All Together

		Chapter
A	**Doing a needs assessment.**	
	Have you:	
1	Included target audience input?	1
2	Included health professional input?	1,4
3	Included other stake holder input?	1
4	Analyzed and synthesized data?	1,2
5	Checked the accuracy of synthesis by sharing your findings with potential participants?	1
B	**Writing program objectives.**	
1	Are there objectives for behavior change?	3
2	Are there objectives for health status change?	3
	Will these behavior changes lead to health status change?	3
3	Are there objectives for teaching methods?	3

4	Are there objectives for attendance?	3
5	Are there means for measuring if the objectives are being met?	2,3
6	Do the objectives reflect the findings of the needs assessments?	1,3

C Preparing an intervention.

1	Do you have a framework based on theory and models?	7
2	Are your content and delivery methods based on your framework?	3,7
3	Have you defined the delivery method (one to one, group, media)?	3
4	Who will deliver the intervention?	3
5	Does the deliverer(s) know what to deliver?	3
6	Does the deliverer(s) have the skills to teach?	3
7	Did the deliverer(s) participate in the design?	1
8	Does the deliverer(s) have the skills to deal with 'problem' patients?	5,6
9	Will the deliverer(s) give the education as designed?	3
10	How much time will patients have?	3
11	How much time can deliverers devote?	3
12	Is space available?	3
13	Are funds available to pay for staff time/space?	3
14	Does the program reflect the findings of the needs assessment?	1,3
15	Will the intervention lead participants to meet the objectives?	3
16	Does the teaching method reflect the use of theory?	3,7
17	Does the teaching reflect the strengths of various teaching methods?	3
18	Is there a detailed written protocol?	3
19	Is the patient education delivered according to the protocol?	2
20	Is the patient education culturally relevant?	4

21	Do patients understand the patient education?	3,4

D Getting patients and program together.

1	Is there a plan for informing potential participants about the program?	4
2	Is the plan functioning?	2
3	Do health professionals refer patients to the program?	2
4	Are the major media involved?	4
5	Are informal information systems involved?	4
6	Is the program time convenient for patients?	4
7	Is the program location convenient for patients?	4
8	Is the program site perceived of as hospitable by patients?	4

E Evaluating patient education programs.

1	Do you know what you want to evaluate?	2
2	Do you have a formal evaluation plan?	2
3	Do you have instruments (questionnaires) to evaluate what you want to evaluate?	2
4	Are the data actually being collected?	2
5	Do you know how to analyze the data?	2
6	Are the data being analyzed?	2
7	Are the evaluation results being used?	2

Now it is your turn. What did you find useful? What did you want to know that was not covered in this book? What practical tips do you have to help others? Please let me know. Needs assessments are an ongoing process. You are the client for this book, so your input is vital. See page xii for my address.

Appendix

Patient Education
Evaluation Scales

This appendix consists of several self-administered questionnaires which have been used in evaluating patient education programs. All of these scales have met all the standard criteria for questionnaires and have been published in national journals. All of these scales can be used without further permission from the authors.

For each scale we have given three pieces of information: (1) the actual scale, (2) information on how to score the scale, and (3) references to how the scale was designed and validated.

The following is an overview of the scales.

1. Visual Analogue Scales for pain and quality of life. These scales are an excellent easy way to measure subject states such as pain, quality of life or stress.
2. The Health Assessment Questionnaire. This scale measures disability. It has been used in the National Health Survey and in many chronic disease studies.
3. The Medical Outcome Studies (MOS) short form was developed by the Rand Corporation and is one of the most promising of the new scales. It measures physical functioning, role functioning, social functioning, pain and health perceptions. You may use any or all of these scales.
4. The Center for Epidemiologic Studies Depression Scale (CES-D) was developed to measure depression in the general population. We like it better than other self-administered depression scales because it is especially sensitive in picking up subclinical depression. This level of depression is very common in people suffering physical disease.
5. The Self-Report Medication Scale is a quick easy way to measure compliance. It was designed for a high blood pressure study. While other means of monitoring compliance, such as laboratory testing, may produce more accurate results, this short easy scale should not be discounted. It does quite well in getting a general idea of what is happening.
6. The Patient Satisfaction Scale is just that, a means of measuring patient satisfaction.

For more information on these scales read the references.

Visual Analogue Scales

Pain Visual Analogue Scale

We are interested in learning whether or not you are affected by pain because of your illness. Please mark an X on the line below to describe your arthritis pain in the *recent past*.

Pain as bad   No

as could be ⊢————————————————————⊣ pain

SEVERE   MODERATE   SLIGHT

Quality of Life Visual Analogue Scale

Take a moment and think of the best possible life and the worst possible life. Now, on the line below, place an X to indicate where your life is *now*.

Worst   Best

possible   possible

life ⊢————————————————————⊣ life

Scoring

Measure in centimeters with ruler, 10 being 'Pain as bad as can be' or 'Worst possible life' and 0 being 'No pain' or 'Best possible life'. Enter the number where the middle of the X is located. Enter whole numbers, not decimals. If the X is between centimeters, round down if below 0.5, round up if 0.5 and above.

Note: The line must be *exactly* 10 cm long. When reproducing, make sure your printer or copy machine reproduces at exactly 100%. (Kodak copiers, for example, generally reproduce at 100%, Xerox doesn't.) You cannot have a reliable measurement if the line isn't exactly the same length each time.

References

1   Dixon, J.S., Bird, H.A.,
   Reproducibility along a 10 cm vertical visual analogue scale, *Annals of the Rheumatic Diseases,* 40:87–89, 1981.

2   Downie, W.W., Leatham, P.A., Rhind, V.A., Wright, V., Branco, J.A., Anderson, J.A.,
     Studies with pain rating scales, *Annals of the Rheumatic Diseases,* 37:378–381, 1978.

3   Downie, W.W., Leatham, P.A., Rhind, V.A., Pickup, M.E., Wright, V.,
     The visual analogue scale in the assessment of grip strength, *Annals of the Rheumatic Diseases,* 37:382–384, 1978.

4   Scott, R.J., Huskisson, E.C.,
     Measurement of functional capacity with visual analogue scales, *Rheumatology and Rehabilitation,* 16:257–259, 1977.

5   Scott, R.J., Huskisson, E.C.,
     Graphic representation of pain. *Pain,* 2:175–184, 1976.

6   Jacobsen, M.,
     The use of rating scales in clinical research. *British Journal of Psychiatry,* 3:545–546, 1965.

Health Assessment Questionnaire (HAQ)

Please check the one response which best describes your usual abilities
OVER THE PAST WEEK:

	Without ANY Difficulty	*With SOME Difficulty*	*With MUCH Difficulty*	*UNABLE to Do*
DRESSING AND GROOMING				
Are you able to:				
Dress yourself, including tying shoelaces and doing buttons?	____	____	____	____
Shampoo your hair?	____	____	____	____
ARISING				
Are you able to:				
Stand up from an armless straight chair?	____	____	____	____
Get in and out of bed?	____	____	____	____
EATING				
Are you able to:				
Cut your meat?	____	____	____	____
Lift a full cup or glass to your mouth?	____	____	____	____
WALKING				
Are you able to:				
Walk outdoors on flat ground?	____	____	____	____
Climb up five steps?	____	____	____	____

• **Please check any AIDS OR DEVICES that you usually use for any of these activities:**

_____	Cane	_____	Devices used for dressing (buttonhook, zipper pull, long-handled shoehorn, etc.)
_____	Walker	_____	Built-up or special utensils
_____	Crutches	_____	Special or built-up chair
_____	Wheelchair	_____	Other (Specify _____)

• **Please check any categories for which you usually need HELP FROM ANOTHER PERSON:**

_____	Dressing and grooming	_____	Eating
_____	Arising	_____	Walking

• **Please check the one response which best describes your usual abilities OVER THE PAST WEEK:**

	Without ANY Difficulty	*With SOME Difficulty*	*With MUCH Difficulty*	*UNABLE to Do*
HYGIENE				
Are you able to:				
Wash and dry your entire body?	_____	_____	_____	_____
Take a tub bath?	_____	_____	_____	_____
Get on and off the toilet?	_____	_____	_____	_____
REACH				
Are you able to:				
Reach and get down a five pound object (such as a bag of sugar) from just above your head?	_____	_____	_____	_____
Bend down to pick up clothing from the floor?	_____	_____	_____	_____
GRIP				
Are you able to:				
Open car doors?	_____	_____	_____	_____
Open jars which have been previously opened?	_____	_____	_____	_____
Turn faucets on and off?	_____	_____	_____	_____

(Continued on next page)

	Without ANY Difficulty	With SOME Difficulty	With MUCH Difficulty	UNABLE to Do

ACTIVITIES

Are you able to:

Run errands and shop? _____ _____ _____ _____

Get in and out of a car? _____ _____ _____ _____

Do chores such as vacuuming
and yardwork? _____ _____ _____ _____

• **Please check any AIDS or DEVICES that you usually use for any of these activities:**

_____ Raised toilet seat _____ Bathtub bar

_____ Bathtub seat _____ Long-handled
appliances for reach

_____ Jar opener (for _____ Long-handled appliances
jars previously in bathroom
opened)

_____ Other (Specify _____)

• **Please check any categories for which you usually need HELP FROM ANOTHER PERSON:**

_____ Hygiene _____ Gripping and opening things

_____ Reach _____ Errands and chores

Scoring

Each of the eight categories (Dressing and Grooming, Arising, Eating, Walking, etc.) are coded as a separate unit. The score for each category is determined by the highest score for *any* of the subquestions in that category.

0 = Without ANY difficulty
1 = With SOME difficulty
2 = With MUCH difficulty
3 = UNABLE to do

Example

	Without ANY Difficulty	*With SOME Difficulty*	*With MUCH Difficulty*	*UNABLE to Do*
HYGIENE				
Are you able to:				
Wash and dry your entire body?	✔	___	___	___
Take a tub bath?	___	✔	___	___
Get on and off the toilet?	✔	___	___	___

This category (hygiene) would be coded as 1.

Each category is coded according to the basic rules. However, if any AIDS OR DEVICES and/or HELP FROM ANOTHER PERSON items listed after each section are checked, the score for the category to which they apply is adjusted upward to 2. If the basic score is **already** 2 or 3, the score remains unchanged. AIDS OR DEVICES and/or HELP FROM ANOTHER PERSON can *only* change a category's score to 2. They *cannot* change the score to a 1 or a 3. The score for the full scale is the average of the 8 category scales. (Add the 8 scores and divide by 8.) The final score is always between 0 and 3.

The categories to which specific devices apply are listed below:

Cane (walking)
Walker (walking)
Crutches (walking)
Wheelchair (walking)
Raised toilet (hygiene)
Bathtub seat (hygiene)
Jar opener (grip)
Devices for dressing (dressing and grooming)
Built-up or special utensils (eating)

Special chair (arising)
Other (judge whether it is a *special* device designed for the task, not something which is used normally by people without disability)
Bathtub bar (hygiene)
Long-handled appliance for reach (reach)
Long-handled appliance for bath (hygiene)

References

Fries, J.F., Spitz, P., Kraines, R.G., Holman, H.R., Measurement of patient outcome in arthritis. *Arthritis and Rheumatism,* 23:137–145, 1980.

The Medical Outcomes Study Short Form (MOS)

1. In general, would you say your health is:

	(Circle *one*)
Excellent	1
Very good	2
Good	3
Fair	4
Poor	5

2. How much *bodily* pain have you generally had during the *past 4 weeks?*

	(Circle *one*)
None	1
Very mild	2
Mild	3
Moderate	4
Severe	5
Very severe	6

3. How much (if at all) has your health limited you in each of the following activities?

(Circle *one* number on each line)

		Yes, limited a lot	*Yes, limited a little*	*No, not limited at all*
a.	The kinds or amounts of vigorous activities you can do, like lifting heavy objects, running, or participating in strenuous sports	1	2	3
b.	The kinds or amounts of moderate activities you can do, like moving a table, carrying groceries or bowling	1	2	3
c.	Walking uphill or climbing a few flights of stairs	1	2	3
d.	Bending, lifting or stooping	1	2	3
e.	Walking one block	1	2	3
f.	Eating, dressing, bathing, or using the toilet	1	2	3

4. Does your health *keep* you from working at a job, doing work around the house or going to school?

    (Circle *one*)

    Yes, for more than three months   1

    Yes, for three months or less   2

    No   3

5. Have you been unable to do *certain kinds* or *amounts* of work, housework or schoolwork because of your health?

    (Circle *one*)

    Yes, for more than three months   1

    Yes, for three months or less   2

    No   3

6. Please circle the number which best describes whether each of the following statements is true or false for you.

    (Circle *one* number on each line)

		Definitely true	*Mostly true*	*Not true*	*Mostly false*	*Definitely false*
a.	I am somewhat ill	1	2	3	4	5
b.	I am as healthy as anybody I know	1	2	3	4	5

7. How often during the *past 4 weeks*

(Circle *one* number on each line)

		All of the time	*Most of the time*	*A good bit of the time*	*Some of the time*	*A little of the time*	*None of the time*
a.	Has your health limited your social activities (like visiting with friends or close relatives)?	1	2	3	4	5	6
b.	Have you been a very nervous person?	1	2	3	4	5	6
c.	Have you felt calm and peaceful?	1	2	3	4	5	6
d.	Have you felt down-hearted and blue?	1	2	3	4	5	6
e.	Have you been a happy person?	1	2	3	4	5	6
f.	Have you felt so down in the dumps that nothing could cheer you up?	1	2	3	4	5	6

8. Please circle the number which best describes whether each of the following statements is true or false for you.

(Circle *one* number on each line)

		Definitely true	*Mostly true*	*Not true*	*Mostly false*	*Definitely false*
a.	My health is excellent	1	2	3	4	5
b.	I have been feeling bad lately	1	2	3	4	5

Scoring

The MOS short form has five subscales: Physical Functioning, Role Functioning, Social Functioning, Health Perceptions and Pain. Scores on each subscale are the sum of the scores for the questions within the subscale. With the exception of Pain, the higher the score, the better. Pain is the opposite; the higher the score, the more pain the person is reporting.

The scores for some questions (1, 6a, 8b, 7c, 7e) must be *reversed* before being calculated. (For example, 1=6, 6=1, 2=5, 5=2, 3=4, 4=3.) Subscales are made up of the following questions:

Physical Functioning:	Questions 3a through 3f
Role Functioning:	Questions 4 and 5
Social Functioning:	Questions 7a through 7f (reverse 7c and 7e)
Health Perceptions:	Questions 1 (reverse), 6a and 6b, 8a and 8b (reverse 6a and 8b)
Pain:	Question 2

If you wish to compare your MOS results with those in other studies using the MOS, you will need to transform the scales. More information on doing this, as well as the handling of missing data, can be found in the article cited below.

References

Stewart, A.L., Hays, R.D., Ware, J.E.,
The MOS short-form general survey: reliability and validity in a patient population, *Medical Care,* 26:724–735, 1988.

The Center for Epidemiologic
Studies Depression Scale (CES-D)

Below is a list of some of the ways you may have felt or behaved. Please indicate how often you have felt this way during the **past week** by checking the appropriate space.

	Rarely or none of the time (less than 1 day)	*Some or a little of the time (1–2 days)*	*Occasionally or a moderate amount of time (3–4 days)*	*All of the time (5–7 days)*
1. I was bothered by things that usually don't bother me.	_____	_____	_____	_____
2. I did not feel like eating; my appetite was poor.	_____	_____	_____	_____
3. I felt that I could not shake off the blues, even with help from my family.	_____	_____	_____	_____
4. I felt that I was just as good as other people.	_____	_____	_____	_____
5. I had trouble keeping my mind on what I was doing.	_____	_____	_____	_____

(Continued on the next page.)

	Rarely or none of the time (less than 1 day)	Some or a little of the time (1–2 days)	Occasion-ally or a moderate amount of time (3–4 days)	All of the time (5–7 days)
6. I felt depressed.	_____	_____	_____	_____
7. I felt that everything I did was an effort.	_____	_____	_____	_____
8. I felt hopeful about the future.	_____	_____	_____	_____
9. I thought my life had been a failure.	_____	_____	_____	_____
10. I felt fearful.	_____	_____	_____	_____
11. My sleep was restless.	_____	_____	_____	_____
12. I was happy.	_____	_____	_____	_____
13. I talked less than usual.	_____	_____	_____	_____
14. I felt lonely.	_____	_____	_____	_____

(Continued on the next page.)

	Rarely or none of the time (less than 1 day)	Some or a little of the time (1–2 days)	Occasion-ally or a moderate amount of time (3–4 days)	All of the time (5–7 days)
15. People were unfriendly.	_____	_____	_____	_____
16. I enjoyed life.	_____	_____	_____	_____
17. I had crying spells.	_____	_____	_____	_____
18. I felt sad.	_____	_____	_____	_____
19. I felt that people disliked me.	_____	_____	_____	_____
20. I could not get going.	_____	_____	_____	_____

Scoring

	Rarely or none of the time (less than 1 day)	Some or a little of the time (1–2 days)	Occasion-ally or a moderate amount of time (3–4 days)	All of the time (5–7 days)
			Item Weights	
1. I was bothered by things that usually don't bother me.	0	1	2	3
2. I did not feel like eating; my appetite was poor.	0	1	2	3
3. I felt that I could not shake off the blues, even with help from my family.	0	1	2	3
4. I felt that I was just as good as other people.	3	2	1	0
5. I had trouble keeping my mind on what I was doing.	0	1	2	3

(Continued on the next page.)

	Rarely or none of the time (less than 1 day)	Some or a little of the time (1–2 days)	Occasion-ally or a moderate amount of time (3–4 days)	All of the time (5–7 days)
			Item Weights	
6. I felt depressed.	0	1	2	3
7. I felt that everything I did was an effort.	0	1	2	3
8. I felt hopeful about the future.	3	2	1	0
9. I thought my life had been a failure.	0	1	2	3
10. I felt fearful.	0	1	2	3
11. My sleep was restless.	0	1	2	3
12. I was happy.	3	2	1	0
13. I talked less than usual.	0	1	2	3

(Continued on the next page.)

	Rarely or none of the time (less than 1 day)	Some or a little of the time (1–2 days)	Occasion-ally or a moderate amount of time (3–4 days)	All of the time (5–7 days)
	Item Weights			
14. I felt lonely.	0	1	2	3
15. People were unfriendly.	0	1	2	3
16. I enjoyed life.	3	2	1	0
17. I had crying spells.	0	1	2	3
18. I felt sad.	0	1	2	3
19. I felt that people disliked me.	0	1	2	3
20. I could not get going.	0	1	2	3

Score is the sum of the twenty item weights. Possible range is 0 to 60. If more than four questions are missing answers, do not score the CES-D. A score of 16 or more is considered depressed.

Reference

Radloff, L.S.,
The CES-D scale: a self-report depression scale for research in the general population. *Applied Psychological Measurement,* 1:385–401, 1977.

—◆—

Self-Reported Medication-Taking Scale

(Circle *one*)

1. Do you ever forget to take your medicine?   Yes   No
2. Are you careless at times about taking
   your medicine   Yes   No
3. When you feel better do you sometimes
   stop taking your medicine?   Yes   No
4. Sometimes if you feel worse when you take
   the medicine, do you stop taking it?   Yes   No

Scoring

This scale is designed to test medication compliance. To score, code Yes = 0, No = 1. The sum of the answers is the score. A score of 4 is considered high comliance, 3 is moderate compliance, 2 or less is low complaince.

Reference

Morisky, D.E., Green, L.W., Levine, D.M.,
Concurrent and predictive validity of a self-reported measure of medication adherence, *Medical Care,* 24:67–74, 1986.

Your Health Care

Thinking about *your own health care,* how would you rate the following?

(Circle one number on each line)

	Poor	Fair	Good	Very Good	Excellent
OVERALL					
1. Overall, how would you evaluate health care at [plan]?	1	2	3	4	5

ACCESS: Arranging for and Getting Care

	Poor	Fair	Good	Very Good	Excellent
2. Convenience of location of the doctor's office	1	2	3	4	5
3. Hours when the doctor's office is open	1	2	3	4	5
4. Access to specialty care if you need it	1	2	3	4	5
5. Access to hospital care if you need it	1	2	3	4	5
6. Access to medical care in an emergency	1	2	3	4	5
7. Arrangements for making appointments for medical care by phone	1	2	3	4	5
8. Length of time spent waiting at the office to see the doctor	1	2	3	4	5

	Poor	Fair	Good	Very Good	Excellent
9. Length of time you wait between making an appointment for routine care and the day of your visit	1	2	3	4	5
10. Availability of medical information or advice by phone	1	2	3	4	5
11. Access to medical care whenever you need it	1	2	3	4	5
12. Services available for getting perscriptions filled	1	2	3	4	5

FINANCES

	Poor	Fair	Good	Very Good	Excellent
13. Protection you have against hardship due to medical expenses	1	2	3	4	5
14. Arrangements for you to get the medical care you need without financial problems	1	2	3	4	5

TECHNICAL QUALITY

	Poor	Fair	Good	Very Good	Excellent
15. Thoroughness of examinations and accuracy of diagnoses	1	2	3	4	5
16. Skill, experience, and training of doctors	1	2	3	4	5
17. Thoroughness of treatment	1	2	3	4	5

	Poor	Fair	Good	Very Good	Excellent

COMMUNICATION

	Poor	Fair	Good	Very Good	Excellent
18. Explanations of medical procedures and tests	1	2	3	4	5
19. Attention given to what you have to say	1	2	3	4	5
20. Advice you get about ways to avoid illness and stay healthy	1	2	3	4	5

CHOICE AND CONTINUITY

	Poor	Fair	Good	Very Good	Excellent
21. Number of doctors you have to choose from	1	2	3	4	5
22. Arrangements for choosing a personal doctor	1	2	3	4	5
23. Ease of seeing the doctor of your choice	1	2	3	4	5

INTERPERSONAL CARE

	Poor	Fair	Good	Very Good	Excellent
24. Friendliness and courtesy shown to you by your doctors	1	2	3	4	5
25. Personal interest in you and your medical problems	1	2	3	4	5
26. Respect shown to you, attention to your privacy	1	2	3	4	5

	Poor	Fair	Good	Very Good	Excellent
27. Reassurance and support offered to you by your doctors and staff	1	2	3	4	5
28. Friendliness and courtesy shown to you by staff	1	2	3	4	5
29. Amount of time you have with doctors and staff during a visit	1	2	3	4	5

OUTCOMES

	Poor	Fair	Good	Very Good	Excellent
30. The outcomes of your medical care, how much you are helped	1	2	3	4	5
31. Overall quality of care and services	1	2	3	4	5

Attitudes Toward Care

Below are some things people say about their medical care. Please read each one carefully, keeping in mind your health care plan. Although the statements may look similar, please answer each one separately.

(Circle one number on each line)

	Strongly agree	Agree	Not sure	Dis-agree	Strongly disagree
32. I am very satisfied with the medical care I receive	1	2	3	4	5
33. There are some things about the medical care I receive that could be better	1	2	3	4	5
34. The medical care I have been receiving is just about perfect	1	2	3	4	5
35. I am dissatisfied with some things about the medical care I receive	1	2	3	4	5

Scoring

For all items except 32 through 34:

    1 = poor
    2 = fair
    3 = good
    4 = very good
    5 = excellent

For items 32 through 34 score as follows:

    1 = 5
    2 = 4
    3 = 4
    4 = 2
    5 = 1

By using the above scoring all items and scales are scored with the higher ratings being best.

You have a choice of using the scores for the individual items or to cluster items (as they are on the questionnaire) into a scale (Access, Finances, Technical Quality, Communications, Choice and Continuity, Interpersonal Care, and Attitudes Toward Care). To score a scale add the score of all the items and divide by the number of items in the scale. This will give you the mean or average scale score.

If half or more of the items are missing, consider the whole scale as missing. Do not count missing items when you are figuring a scale score.

Please note: The complete GHAA's Consumer Satisfaction Survey contains a number of additional scales for rating one's health insurance plan. The reference for the complete survey and the user's manual is given below.

Reference

Davies, A.R., Ware, J.E.,
GHHA's Consumer Satisfaction Survey and User's Manual (second edition), Department of Research and Analysis, Group Health Association of America, Inc., 1129 Twentieth St., NW, Suite 600, Washington, DC, 20036, 1991.

Index

A

Activities, protocols for, 49, 50–51
Activity, as coping strategy, 121
Advertising, media for, 74
AIDS, 7, 119, 130
Alcoholics Anonymous, 111
American Cancer Society Reach for
Recovery program, 114
Antagonism, by patient, 88
Appraisal, 118–19
Arthritis
in elderly, 71
exercise for, 95, 97
language describing, 97, 116
types of, 57–58
Arthritis program, rural, 40
Arthritis Self-Help Course, 114
protocol from, 50–63
Asthma, self-monitoring of, 45
Attention-seeking patient, 89–90
Avoidance, 121

B

Back pain, 121
Behavior change
compliance and, 95
enabling factors for, 128
reinforcing factors for, 128–29
Behavior program, self-directed, 31, 33
Behavior(s)
complex, 98–99
contracts for, 111, 112–14
determining effectiveness of, 32–33
easily changeable, 33
listing, 32
modeling, 114–16
Beliefs
changing, 127
salient, assessment of, 5–7
Belligerence, by patient, 88

Biased patients, 90
Brainstorming, 41–42, 85–86
Breast examination, 46
Breast lump, 118–19

C

Cardiac patients, evaluation of compliance by, 18–19
Cardiac rehabilitation education, 7
Center for Epidemiologic Studies
Depression Scale, 145, 159–64
Charts, for arthritis course, 53–54, 59, 60
Checklist
for education program, 139–41
for needs assessment, 5
Children
handicapped, 18
needs of, 4
Cholesterol, lowering, 31, 32–33
Coaching, 42
Community resources, 78–81
Comparisons, in evaluations, 25–26
Compliance, 95–103
belief in skills for, 100–101
belief in value of, 97
decision chart for, 102
importance of, 96
patient understanding and, 97–98
reason for lack of, 96
skill required for, 98–100
undesired, 101
Computer, questionnaires on, 11
Computer based education, (CBE), 38–39
Confronting, 119–20
Contracts, for behavior, 111, 112–14
Coping theory, 117–22
Costs, 72–73
Cultural groups, needs of, 3

O

Objectives
  applied to program planning, 36–37
  types of, 34–35
  writing, 35–36
Opinion leaders, 69, 76–77
Outcome evaluation, 17
Outcome objectives, 35, 37

P

Pain, 97, 121
Patients
  hard to help (see Difficult patients)
  hard to reach, 75–78
Patient Satisfaction Scale, 145, 166–70
Perceived threats, 130–31
Persuasion, of patients, 116–17
Physical capacity, for skills learning,
  100
Place for education program, 73
Planning and implementation, 31–64
  group education, 49
  one to one education, 46–49
  problems with groups, 31
  process, 37–46
  protocols, 49–63
  setting objectives, 34–37
  setting priorities, 31–34
Prayer, 122
PRECEDE model, 126–29, 130
Printed materials, 40
Problem solving, as coping behavior,
  121
Process evaluation, 17
Process objectives, 34–35, 37
Protocols, 49–63
Public, marketing to, 71–73
Publicity, 74. *See also* Marketing;
  Networking
Punishment, from compliance, 98

Q

Qualitative evaluations, 17–19
Quantitative evaluations, 19–25
Questioning, in patient teaching, 43–44
Questionnaire(s)
  on computer, 11
  design of, 20
  for interested party analysis, 4
  pitfalls, 21–24
  for salient beliefs assessment, 6
  self-administered, for program
   evaluation, 145–70
Questions
  for brainstorming, 41
  wording of, 19

R

Radio, advertising on, 74
Randomized design, 25–26
Reach for Recovery program, 114
Reappraisal, positive, 121
Referrals, 70
Rehearsal, 43
Reinforcement, 128–29
Responsibility, accepting, 120–121
Rewards, for compliance, 98
Role playing, 42

S

Salient beliefs assessment, 5–7
Scripts, for arthritis course, 61–62
Self-control, 120
Self-Report Medication Scale, 145, 165
Skills mastery, 111
Smoking, 18, 24, 34, 46, 123
Social support, 120
Software, for questionnaires, 11
Stanford Heart Diseases Prevention
  Project, 38
Statements, self-, 122, 125
Statistics, 24–25